Atul Gawande

Biography

The Journey of a Surgeon and Innovator

CONTENT

Part I: Fallibility

Chapter 1: Education of a Knife

Chapter 2: The Computer and the Hernia Factory

Chapter 3: When Doctors Make Mistakes

Chapter 4: Nine Thousand Surgeons

Chapter 5: When Good Doctors Go Bad

Part II: Mystery

Chapter 6: Full Moon Friday the Thirteenth

Chapter 7: The Pain Perplex

Chapter 8: A Queasy Feeling

Chapter 9: Crimson Tide

Chapter 10: The Man Who Couldn't Stop Eating

Part III: Uncertainty

Chapter 11: Final Cut

Chapter 12: The Dead Baby Mystery

Chapter 13: Whose Body Is It, Anyway?

Chapter 14: The Case of the Red Leg

Part 1: Fallibility

Chapter 1: Education of a knife

This was my fourth week of surgical training. My short white coat's pockets were bulging with patient printouts, laminated cards with CPR and dictation system instructions, two surgical handbooks, a stethoscope, wound-dressing supplies, lunch tickets, a penlight, scissors, and approximately a $1 in change. As I walked up the stairs to the patient's floor, I rattled.

This will be good, I tried to convince myself: my first genuine surgery. My patient—fiftyish, thick, and taciturn—was recovering from abdominal surgery he had had about a week prior. His digestive function had not yet recovered, therefore he was unable to eat. I explained to him that he needed intravenous feeding, which required a "special line" that would be inserted into his chest. I explained that I would insert the line while he was on his bed, lying him flat, numbing a place on his chest with local anesthesia, and then threading the line in. I didn't mention that the line was eight inches long and would enter his vena cava, the main blood vessel to his heart. Nor did I mention how difficult the surgery would be. I stated that there were "slight risks" involved, such as hemorrhage or lung collapse; under expert hands, such complications occur in less than one out of every hundred cases.

Once the tip of this needle is in the vein, you must widen the hole in the vein wall, insert the catheter, and thread it in the correct direction—down to the heart rather than up to the brain—without tearing through any veins, lungs, or other structures. To do this, S. indicated that you must first install a guidewire. She removed the syringe, leaving the needle in place. Blood flowed out. She took a two-foot-long twenty-gauge wire that resembled an electric guitar's steel D string and threaded it almost entirely through the needle's bore, into the vein, and onward toward the vena cava. "Never force it in," she said, "and never ever let go of it." The cardiac monitor displayed a series of fast heartbeats, prompting her to hurriedly pull the wire back an inch. She removed the needle from the wire and replaced it with a bullet of thick, rigid plastic, which she pressed in tightly to expand the vein opening. She next withdrew the dilator and ran the central line—a spaghetti-thick, yellow, flexible plastic tube—over the wire until it was fully inserted. She could now remove the cable. She irrigated the line with heparin, then sutured it to his chest. And that was all.

I set the items on a bedside table, unfastened the patient's gown behind his neck, and positioned him flat on the mattress, chest bare and arms at his sides. I turned on a bright overhead light and adjusted his bed to my height. I summoned S. to come. I put on my gown and gloves and placed out the central line, guidewire, and other kit components on a sterile tray, just as S. had done. I drew five cc of lidocaine into a syringe, soaked two sponge sticks in the yellow-brown Betadine antiseptic solution, and opened the suture package. I was fine to go.

She let me proceed with the next steps, which I stumbled through. I didn't know how long and floppy the guidewire was until I drew it out of its plastic cover and inserted one end into the patient, almost letting the other touch his unsterile bedsheet. I'd forgotten about the dilating stage until she reminded me. Then, when I put in the dilator, I didn't push hard enough, so S. pushed it all the way in. Finally, we inserted the line, flushed it, and sutured it in place. Outside the room, S. suggested that I be less tentative the next time, but that I shouldn't be too concerned about how things went.The method remained completely mysterious to me. And I couldn't get over the thought of inserting a needle so deeply and blindly into someone's chest. I anticipated the X-ray with apprehension. But everything came back fine: I had not harmed the lung, and the line was in the proper location.

Not everyone enjoys the benefits of surgery. When you first enter the operating room as a medical student and see the surgeon apply the scalpel to someone's body and open it like fruit, you either tremble in fear or gape in amazement. I gaped. It wasn't simply the blood and intestines that captivated me. The notion was that a normal person would have the confidence to use that scalpel in the first place. Later, while still a student, I was permitted to make an incision myself. The surgeon used a marking pen to draw a six-inch dotted line over a sleeping patient's belly before handing me the knife, which surprised me. It was still warm from the autoclave, as far as I remember. The surgeon instructed me to use my free hand's thumb and forefinger to stretch the skin taut. He instructed me to make a single smooth slice down to the fat. I applied the belly of the blade to the skin and cut. The experience was strange and addictive, combining excitement from the controlled ferocity of the act, worry about getting it perfect, and a righteous belief that it was somehow beneficial to the individual. There was also the slightly unpleasant feeling of discovering that it required more force than I had anticipated. (The skin is thick and elastic, and on my first pass, I did not go deep enough; I had to cut twice to go through.) The scene made me want to be a surgeon—not just an amateur with a knife for a little while, but someone with the confidence to proceed as if it were regular.

A resident, on the other hand, begins with no sense of mastery—only an overwhelming desire to avoid doing anything like pushing a knife against flesh or jabbing a needle into someone's chest. On my first day as a surgical resident, I was assigned to the ER. One of my first patients was a slender, dark-haired woman in her late twenties who staggered in, teeth gritted, with a two-and-a-half-foot-long wooden chair leg mysteriously attached to the bottom of her foot. She claimed that the leg had collapsed from under a kitchen chair she had attempted to sit on, and when leaping up to avoid falling, she accidently stamped her bare foot on the three-inch screw protruding out of it. I worked really hard to look like someone who hadn't just received his medical diploma the week before. Instead, I was resolved to be unconcerned, world-weary, the type of guy who had seen this a hundred times before. I examined her foot and discovered that the screw was embedded in the bone near the base of her big toe. There was no blood and, as far as I could tell, no fracture.

The logical thing to do was give her a tetanus shot and remove the screw. I purchased the tetanus injection, but I began to have reservations about removing the screw. Suppose she bled? Or perhaps I shattered her foot? Or something worse? I excused myself and sought out Dr. W, the senior surgeon on duty. I discovered him ministering to a car accident victim. The patient was a mess. Everyone was shouting. There was blood all over the floor. It was not the best time to ask questions. I ordered an X-ray. I felt it would buy time and allow me to confirm my amateur impression that she did not have a fracture.

Finally, I made myself do it. I gave her a one-two-three and pulled, first gingerly and then fiercely. She moaned. The screw wouldn't budge. I twisted, and it suddenly came free. There was no blood. I cleansed the wound as my textbooks instructed for puncture wounds. She discovered she could walk, despite her hurting foot. I informed her about the dangers of infection and what symptoms to look for. Her appreciation was enormous and flattering, like the lion's for the mouse—and that night I went home ecstatic. Skill and confidence in surgery, like in any other field, are acquired via painful and humiliating experience. We, like the tennis player, the oboist, and the guy who fixes hard drives, must practice in order to become proficient in our craft. However, there is one difference in medicine: we practice on individuals.

Despite this, the operation proved ineffective. I stuck the needle too shallowly, then too deeply. Frustration overcame hesitancy, and I attempted one angle after another. Nothing worked. Then, for a brief period, I saw a flare of blood in the syringe, signaling that I had entered the vein. I anchored the needle with one hand and pulled the syringe with the other. However, the syringe was too securely attached, so when I pulled it free, the needle was released from the vein. The patient started leaking into her chest wall. I applied pressure as best I could for five minutes, but her chest remained black and blue around the location. The hematoma rendered it impossible to run a line through there anymore. I wanted to give up. But she wanted a line, and the resident monitoring me—a second-year this time—was determined that I would succeed. After an X-ray revealed that I had not harmed her lung, he had me try again on the opposite side using a completely new outfit. I still missed, though, and before I could turn the patient into a pincushion, he grabbed control. It took him several minutes and two or three sticks to locate the vein, which made me feel better. Perhaps she was an especially tough case.

When I failed with a third patient a few days later, doubts began to set in. Again, there was stick, stick, and nothing. I stood aside. The resident who was observing me got it on the very next try.

Surgeons, as a group, exhibit an unusual equality. They believe in practice over skill. People frequently believe that you must have excellent hands to become a surgeon, but this is not true. When I interviewed for surgery programs, no one made me sew, do a dexterity test, or make sure my hands were steady. You don't even need all ten fingers to get approved. To be sure, talent helps. Professors remark that every two or three years, they see someone exceptionally gifted graduate from a program—someone who learns up complex manual skills extraordinarily rapidly, sees the operating field as a whole, and detects trouble before it occurs. Nonetheless, attending surgeons believe that what matters most to them is finding people who are conscientious, industrious, and stubborn enough to practice this one difficult thing day and night for years. One surgery professor told me that if he had to choose between a Ph.D. who had painstakingly cloned a gene and a skilled sculptor, he would always go with the Ph.D. Sure, he added, he'd bet on the sculpture being more physically gifted; nevertheless, he'd bet on the Ph.D. being less "flaky." And, ultimately, that is more important. Surgeons think that skills can be taught, but persistence cannot. It's an unusual method to recruitment, yet it persists all the way up the ranks, including in top surgery departments. They pick minions with no surgical skills, train them for years, and then hire the majority of their professors from the same domestic ranks.

And it works. There have been several studies of exceptional performers—international violinists, chess grand masters, professional ice skaters, mathematicians, and so on—and the most significant difference researchers have discovered between them and poorer performers is the cumulative amount of conscious practice they've had. Indeed, the most significant talent may be the ability to practice itself. According to K. Anders Ericsson, a cognitive psychologist and performance expert, the most essential function that intrinsic variables may play is in one's willingness to engage in persistent training. He discovered that elite achievers, like everyone else, loathe practicing. (This is why, for example, athletes and musicians typically stop practicing after they retire.) But, unlike others, they have the determination to persevere.

The circumstances were bad. It was late in the day, and I had been awake all night. The patient was severely obese and weighed more than 300 pounds. He couldn't bear lying flat since the weight of his chest and abdomen made it difficult for him to breathe. However, he absolutely required a center line. He had a critically infected wound that required intravenous antibiotics, but no one could find veins in his arms to place a peripheral IV. I had little chance of success. But a resident does as he is told, and I was instructed to attempt the line. I went over my preparations: checking the laboratories, setting out the kit, positioning the towel roll, and so on. I swabbed and draped his chest while he was still sitting upright. S., the chief resident, was watching me this time, and when everything was done, I told her to tip him back with an oxygen mask on his face. His flesh rolled up his chest, like a wave. I couldn't find his clavicle with my fingertips to align the proper place of entry. And he was already looking out of breath, his face flushing. I gave S. the "Do you want to take over?" look. Keep going, she instructed. I took a rough estimate as to where the appropriate location was, numbed it with lidocaine, and then inserted the large needle. For a while, I feared it wouldn't be long enough to fit through, but then I felt the tip slip beneath his clavicle. I pushed a little deeper and pulled back on the syringe. It was unbelievably full of blood. I was in. As I pulled the syringe off and threaded the guidewire in, I concentrated on keeping the needle securely in place and not moving it even a millimeter. The cable went in neatly. He was struggling for air now. We sat him up and let him to regain his breath. Then, after one additional lie-down, I dilated the entry and inserted the central line. S. simply responded, "Nice job," and then went.

Surgical training is the repetition of this process—the flailing, followed by fragments, followed by knowledge, and, on occasion, a moment of elegance—for ever more difficult tasks with ever higher risks. At first, you learn the fundamentals: how to glove and gown, drape patients, grip the knife, and tie a square knot in a length of silk suture (not to mention how to dictate, use computers, and order medicines). However, the chores get more daunting: how to cut through skin, use electrocautery, open the breast, tie off a bleeding vessel, extract the tumor, and heal the wound—a breast lumpectomy. By the end of six months, I'd performed lines, appendectomies, skin grafts, hernia repairs, and mastectomies. At the end of the year, I was performing limb amputations, lymph node biopsies, and hemorrhoidectomies. At the end of two years, I had performed tracheotomies, a few small-bowel operations, and laparoscopic gallbladder surgeries.

I'm in my seventh year of training. Only now does a simple incision through skin appear to be nothing more than the beginning of a case. When I'm inside, the struggle continues. These days, I'm trying to learn how to repair abdominal aortic aneurysms, remove pancreatic cancer, and open blocked carotid artery. I discovered that I am neither brilliant nor maladroit. With more practice, I'll get the hang of it. None of this is exactly false. The attending is in command, and a resident knows better than to forget this. Consider the surgery I performed recently to remove a 75-year-old woman's colon cancer. The attendant stood across from me from the outset. And he, not I, determined where to cut, how to isolate the malignancy, and how much colon to remove.

In medicine, we have long struggled with the requirement to offer the best possible treatment to patients while also providing novices with experience. Residencies try to reduce possible harm through supervision and graduated responsibility. There is grounds to believe that patients benefit from teaching. According to most studies, teaching hospitals outperform non-teaching hospitals. Residents may be inexperienced, but having them around to check on patients, ask questions, and keep professors on their toes appears to help. However, there is no getting past the first few wobbly attempts a young practitioner makes to insert a central line, remove a breast malignancy, or suture two segments of colon. No matter how many safeguards we put in place, these circumstances are typically handled more poorly by novices than experienced individuals.

My sister and I grew up in the little town of Athens, Ohio, where both of our parents are doctors. My mother decided to practice pediatrics part-time, only three half-days a week, because my father's urology practice had grown so busy and successful. He's been doing it for over 25 years, and his office is cluttered with evidence of it: an overflowing wall of patient files, gifts from people displayed everywhere (books, paintings, ceramics with biblical sayings, hand-painted paperweights, blown glass, and carved boxes, as well as a figurine of a boy who pees on you when you pull his pants down). A few dozen of the thousands of kidney stones he has extracted from his patients are stored in an acrylic container beneath his oak desk.

Only now, as I approach the end of my training, have I began to seriously consider my father's achievement. For the most of my residency, I viewed surgery as a more or less fixed body of knowledge and expertise that is learned in training and refined via practice. There was, as I imagined, a smooth, upward-sloping arc of proficiency at some rarefied set of activities (for me, gallbladders, colon tumors, bullets, and appendices; for him, kidney stones, testicular malignancies, and swollen prostates). The area would peak at about 10 or fifteen years, plateau for a long time, and possibly taper off little in the final five years before retirement. The truth, however, proves to be significantly messier. My father says that you get skilled at certain things, but as soon as you do, you realize that what you know is out of date. New technology and operations arise to replace the old, and the learning process begins all over again. "Three-quarters of what I do today I never learned in residency," adds the physician. He has had to learn to put in penile prostheses, perform microsurgery, reverse vasectomies, do nerve-sparing prostatectomies, and implant artificial urinary sphincters on his own, fifty miles away from his nearest colleague—let alone a doctor who could tell him anything like "You need to turn your wrist more when you do that." He's had to learn how to utilize shock-wave lithotripters, electrohydraulic lithotripters, and laser lithotripters (all tools for breaking up kidney stones); to deploy Double J ureteral stents and Silicone Four coil stents and retro-inject multi-length stents (don't even ask) are used to manipulate fiber-optic ureteroscopes. Since he completed his training, he has been introduced to all of these technology and approaches. Some of the procedures were based on past skills. Many didn't.

This is the experience that all surgeons have. The speed of medical innovation has been unstoppable, leaving surgeons with no choice but to attempt new things. Failure to adopt new techniques would deny patients significant medical advances. However, the risks of the learning curve are unavoidable, both in practice and during residency. Patients eventually benefit—often significantly—but the first few patients may not, and may even be damaged. Consider the incident described by the pediatric surgical unit of London's renowned Great Ormond Street Hospital, as detailed in the British Medical Journal in the spring of 2000. The doctors published their findings after operating on 325 consecutive babies with a serious heart defect known as transposition of the great arteries from 1978 to 1998, during which time their surgeons switched from doing one procedure for the condition to another. Such children are born with their heart's outflow vessels reversed: the aorta emerges from the right side of the heart instead of the left, and the artery supplying the lungs exits from the left rather than the right. As a result, blood that enters the body is pumped directly back out rather of being oxygenated in the lungs. This is unsurvivable. The babies perished blue, exhausted, never knowing what it meant to have enough breath.

Then, in the 1980s, a succession of technological improvements enabled safe switch operation. It quickly became the preferred procedure. The Great Ormond Street surgeons made the shift in 1986, and their study demonstrates that it was certainly a positive change. The annual death rate following a successful switch treatment was less than a quarter that of the Senning, resulting in a life expectancy of sixty-three years rather than forty-seven. But the cost of learning to do it was exorbitant. In their first seventy swap surgeries, the surgeons recorded a 25% surgical fatality rate, compared to only 6% with the Senning surgery. (Eighteen newborns died, more than twice the number throughout the entire Senning era.)

They only mastered it over time: only five babies died during their next hundred changeover surgeries.

Recently, a group of Harvard Business School professors who specialize in analyzing learning curves in industry—in semiconductor manufacturing, airplane construction, and so on—decided to investigate learning curves among surgeons. They followed eighteen heart surgeons and their staff as they tried out the novel technique of minimally invasive cardiac surgery. This study, I was startled to learn, is the first of its type. Learning is omnipresent in medicine, but no one has ever compared how well various physicians perform it. The new heart procedure, which involved a little incision between the ribs rather than a chest ripped open down the center, was far more difficult than the standard one. Because the incision is too small to accommodate the standard tubes and clamps for rerouting blood to the heart-bypass machine, doctors had to learn a more difficult approach that utilized balloons and catheters inserted into groin vessels. They had to learn how to operate in considerably smaller spaces. Nurses, anesthesiologists, and perfusionists all had new responsibilities to fulfill. Everyone had new responsibilities, new tools, new ways for things to go wrong, and new methods to correct them. As expected, everyone faced a significant learning curve. Whereas a completely proficient team takes three to six hours for such surgeries, these teams took three times as long for their initial cases. The researchers were unable to track morbidity rates in detail, but it would be stupid to assume that they were unaffected.

The Harvard Business School study provided some encouraging news. We may make significant improvements to the learning curve by being more thoughtful about how we train and track progress, whether with students, residents, or experienced surgeons and nurses. But the study's other findings are less encouraging. No matter how accomplished, surgeons trying something new became worse before they got better, and the learning curve turned out to be longer and more involved than anyone had anticipated. It's all clear evidence that you can't train novices without sacrificing patient care.

One reason I doubt we could sustain a medical training system based on people saying "Yes, you can practice on me" is because I, too, have said no. Walker, my firstborn kid, went into congestive heart failure on a Sunday morning at the age of eleven days due to a major cardiac abnormality. His aorta was not inverted, but a large portion of it had stopped growing completely. My wife and I were terrified—his kidneys and liver had also begun to fail—but he made it to surgery, the repair was successful, and, despite his unpredictable recovery, he was ready to return home after two and a half weeks.

We were far from home free, though. He was born weighing six pounds or more, but at one month old, he weighed only five pounds and would require strict monitoring to ensure that he gained weight. He was on two cardiac drugs that needed to be weaned. And, in the long run, the physicians warned us, his repair would prove inadequate. As Walker developed, his aorta would need to be dilated with a balloon or replaced completely in surgery. They were unable to predict when or how many such procedures would be required over time. A pediatric cardiologist would need to closely monitor him before making a decision.

We hadn't decided who would be our cardiologist as we approached discharge. Walker was treated in the hospital by a large team of cardiologists, including fellows in specialty training and attendings who had been practicing for decades. The day before discharge, one of the young men approached me, presenting his card and suggesting an appointment time for Walker to visit him. He was the team member who had dedicated the most time to caring for Walker. He was the one who saw Walker when we brought him in, inexplicably short of breath, made the diagnosis, got Walker the medications that stabilized him, coordinated with the surgeons, and came to visit us every day to answer our questions. Furthermore, I knew fellows always received their patients in this manner. Most families are unaware of the tiny differences between players, and after a team has saved their child's life, they accept whatever appointment they are given.

I understand this was not fair. My son had an odd difficulty. The fellow needs the experience. I, the inhabitant, should have understood. But I wasn't split on the decision. This was my child. Given the option, I will always provide the greatest care for him. How can anyone be expected to behave otherwise? Certainly, the future of medicine should not be based on it.

The benefit of this coldhearted apparatus extends beyond the fact that it facilitates learning. If learning is vital yet causes harm, it should apply to everyone equally. When given a choice, people wriggle out, and those options are not distributed equitably. They belong to the well-connected and knowledgeable, to insiders rather than outsiders, to the doctor's child but not the truck driver's. If choice cannot be given to everyone, perhaps it is best not to allow it at all. It is 2 p.m. I'm in the intensive care unit. A nurse informed me that Mr. G's central line had clotted. Mr. G has been with us for over a month now. He is in his late sixties, from South Boston, gaunt and tired, hanging on by a thread—or a line, to be accurate. He has multiple holes in his small bowel that surgery has failed to repair, and the bilious contents leak out onto his skin from two little reddish openings in his abdomen's concavity. His only option is to be fed via vein and wait for the fistulae to heal. He requires a new central line.

There is a junior resident on the service. She'd only done one or two lines before. I tell her about Mr. G. I ask her if she's available to do a new line. She misinterprets it as an inquiry. She claims she still has patients to see and a case coming up later. Could I do the line? I tell her no. She can't help but grimace. She is burdened, as I was, and she may be afraid, as I was afraid. When I make her talk through the steps, she begins to focus—it's like a dry run, I suppose. She completes nearly all of the stages, but she forgets to check the labs and about Mr. G's severe allergy to heparin, which is used in the flush for the line. I make certain she registers this, then instruct her to get set up and page me.

The junior resident selects a site for the stick. The patient is frighteningly thin. I see every rib and worry she'll puncture his lung. She injects the numbing medicine. Then she inserts the large needle, and the angle seems completely wrong. I motion for her to reposition. This simply increases her uncertainty. She presses deeper, and I know she doesn't have it. She pulls back on the syringe: no blood. She withdraws the needle and tries again. Again, the angle appears incorrect. This time, Mr. G feels the jab and jerks in pain. I grab his arm. She offers him more numbing medicine. It's everything I can do not to take control. But she can't learn without doing, I remind myself. I decide to give her one more try.

Chapter 2: The Computer and the Hernia Factory

On a summer day in 1996, Hans Ohlin, the fifty-year-old chief of coronary care at the University of Lund Hospital in Sweden, sat in his office with a stack of two thousand two hundred and forty electrocardiograms. Each test result was represented by a sequence of wavy lines flowing from left to right across a letter-size page of graph paper. Ohlin read them alone in his office, so as not to be disturbed. He read them quickly but carefully, one at a time, categorizing them into two piles based on whether he believed the patient was undergoing a heart attack at the time the electrocardiogram (EKG) was taken. To avoid fatigue and inattention, he worked on the EKGs over the course of a week, sorting them in shifts of no more than two hours and taking long breaks. He didn't want any thoughtless errors; the stakes were too high. This was the medical equivalent of the Deep Blue chess match, and Ohlin was cardiology's Gary Kasparov. He faced off against a computer.

EKGs appear overly difficult to medical students at first. An EKG typically includes twelve leads, each of which provides a unique tracing on the printout. However, students are taught to identify a dozen or more features in these tracings, each of which is labeled alphabetically: for example, the downstroke at the start of a beat (the Q wave), the upstroke at the peak of heart contraction (the R wave), the subsequent downstroke (the S wave), and the rounded wave right after the beat (the T wave). Sometimes little changes build up to a heart attack, and sometimes they don't. As a medical student, I learned to decode the EKG as if it were a sophisticated equation. My classmates and I would carry laminated cards in our white lab coat pockets with a list of arcane instructions: calculate the heart rate and the axis of electrical flow, check for a rhythm disturbance, then check for an ST-segment elevation greater than one millimeter in leads V1 to V4, or poor R-wave progression (indicating one type of heart attack), and so on.

Managing all of this information becomes easier with practice, just as drawing a line becomes easier. The learning curve applies equally to diagnosis and technique. An skilled cardiologist may occasionally detect a heart attack with a glance, just as a kid might recognize his mother across a room. However, the test remains persistently obscure. According to studies, between 2 and 8% of patients with heart attacks seen in emergency rooms are incorrectly discharged, with a quarter of these persons dying or suffering a full cardiac arrest. Even if such individuals are not mistakenly discharged, critical care may be delayed if an EKG is misread. Human judgment, including experienced human judgment, falls well short of assurance. The rationale for teaching a computer to interpret an EKG is thus quite compelling. If the results show even a tiny increase in human performance, hundreds of lives could be spared each year.

In 1990, William Baxt, an emergency physician at the University of California at San Diego, published an influential article describing how a "artificial neural network"—a type of computer architecture—could make sophisticated clinical decisions. Such expert systems learn from experience in the same way that humans do: by taking feedback from each success and failure to improve their guesses. In a subsequent study, Baxt demonstrated that a computer could easily outperform a group of clinicians in diagnosing heart attacks among patients with chest pain. However, two-thirds of the physicians in his study were novice residents, who are likely to struggle with EKGs. Can a computer outperform an experienced specialist?

This was the question the Swedish study sought to solve. The investigation was led by Lars Edenbrandt, Ohlin's medical colleague and artificial intelligence expert. Edenbrandt spent five years perfecting his system, first in Scotland and later in Sweden. He gave his computer EKGs from over ten thousand patients, instructing it which ones resembled heart attacks and which did not, until the machine became excellent at deciphering even the most ambiguous EKGs. Then he approached Ohlin, a famous cardiologist in Sweden who reads up to ten thousand EKGs per year. Edenbrandt chose two thousand two hundred and forty EKGs from the hospital files to test both of them on, and exactly half, eleven hundred and twenty, were found to show heart attacks. The results were released quietly in the fall of 1997. Ohlin correctly selected six hundred and twenty. The computer detected seven hundred and thirty-eight. Machine outperformed man by 20%.

As a first-year surgical resident, I learnt how to do a pretty easy surgical procedure: hernia repair. A hernia is a weakness of the abdominal wall, typically in the groin, that permits the abdomen's contents to bulge through. In most hospitals, correcting it—pushing the bulge back in and mending the abdominal wall—takes around 90 minutes and can cost up to $4,000. In 10-15% of cases, the operation fails and the hernia returns. However, none of these figures apply to the Shouldice Hospital, a tiny medical center west of Toronto. Hernia procedures at Shouldice typically last between thirty and forty-five minutes. Their recurrence rate is an amazing 1%. And an operation costs approximately half as much as it does elsewhere. There's arguably no finer place in the world to have your hernia fixed. On a chilly Monday morning, I dressed in a green cotton scrub top and slacks, a disposable mask, and a paper cap and walked among the cases in the Shouldice Hospital's five operating rooms. To describe one case means describing all of them: I observed three surgeons operate on six patients, and none varied from their normal procedure.

In a tiled, box-like operating room, I gazed over the shoulder of Richard Sang, a fifty-one-year-old surgeon with a dry wit and a youthful appearance. Though we chatted during the procedure, Dr. Sang completed each step without pause, almost absently, with the assistant knowing exactly which tissues to retract and the nurse handing over the correct equipment; instructions were absolutely superfluous. The patient, a charming, surprisingly composed guy of around thirty-five, occasionally spoke up from behind the draperies to inquire how things were going. He lay on the table, his lower belly exposed and painted yellow with a bactericidal iodine solution. A plum-sized protrusion was observed on the left side of the pubic bone. Dr. Sang injected local anesthetic into the skin in a diagonal line from the top of the man's left hip to the pubis, following the crease of the groin. With a No. 10 blade, he slashed this line in a single downstroke, revealing golden, glistening fat underneath. The assistant pressed a cloth against each side of the wound to absorb the minor bleeding before pulling it open.

Sang quickly cut through the abdomen wall's outer muscle layer, revealing the spermatic cord, a half-inch cable of blood and spermatic arteries. The patient's bulge, we discovered, was caused by a weakening in the muscle wall beneath the cord, which is a common site. Sang halted down for a moment, meticulously examining for another hernia around the point where the cord entered the inner abdominal wall. Sure enough, he discovered a minor, second hernia—one that, if ignored, would almost probably have resulted in a recurrence. He then ripped open the remaining muscle layers underneath the chord, exposing the entire abdominal wall and pushing the swelling contents back within. If you have a tear in a couch cushion with filling coming through, you can repair it with a patch or by sewing it back together. At my hospital, we normally push the hernia back in, cover it with a durable plastic-like mesh, and suture it to the surrounding tissue. It delivers consistent reinforcement, and the strategy is simple to apply. But Sang, like the other Shouldice surgeons I spoke with, dismissed the idea: they saw the mesh as a risk of infection (since it's a foreign body), expensive (because it can cost hundreds of dollars), and unneeded (because they obtain enviable outcomes without it).

As Sang and I discussed possible alternatives, he sewed the wall back together in three separate muscle layers with tiny wire, ensuring that the edges of each layer overlapped like a double-breasted suit. After Sang closed the patient's skin with little clips and withdrew the draperies, he threw his legs over the table, stood up, and walked out. The surgery had just taken half an hour.

Many surgeons use Shouldice's unique repair procedure but have average recurrence rates. Shouldice's success is due to more than just his technique. Shouldice's doctors perform hernia repairs in the same way that Intel manufactures chips: they refer to themselves as a "focused factory." Even the hospital is specifically created for hernia sufferers. Their rooms lack phones and televisions, and their meals are served in a downstairs dining hall; as a result, the patients are forced to get up and walk around, avoiding diseases linked with inactivity such as pneumonia or leg clots.

After leaving the patient with a nurse, Sang found the next patient and led him back into the operating room. Only three minutes had passed, and the room was already spotless. Fresh sheets and new instruments had already been laid out. And thus the next case started. I asked Byrnes Shouldice, the clinic's founder's son and a hernia surgeon, if he ever got bored doing hernias all day. "No," he said in a Spock-like voice. "Perfection is the excitement."

Although the medical establishment has beginning to acknowledge that automation, such as the Shouldice's, has the potential to improve medical treatment outcomes, many doctors remain skeptical. They have been especially hesitant to apply the same knowledge to medical diagnoses. Most clinicians believe that diagnosis cannot be reduced to a set of generalizations, or a "cookbook," as some call it. Instead, they contend that it must take into consideration the unique characteristics of each patient.

One weekend on duty, I saw a 39-year-old woman with discomfort in her right-lower abdomen who did not fit the appendicitis pattern. She stated that she was fairly comfortable, with no fever or nausea. She was hungry, and she did not react when I pressed on her abdomen. Her test results were mostly inconclusive. However, I continued to advocate appendectomy to the attending surgeon. Her white blood cell count was elevated, indicating illness, and she appeared sick to me. Sick patients can have a distinct appearance that you learn to identify after a while in residency. You may not know what's going on, but you're certain it's something serious. The attending physician accepted my diagnosis, operated, and discovered appendicitis. Not long after, I saw a sixty-five-year-old patient with nearly the same narrative. The lab results were the same; I also received an abdominal scan, which was inconclusive. The patient did not meet the pattern for appendicitis, although he appeared to have it. During surgery, however, the appendix was found to be normal. He developed diverticulitis, which is a colon infection that normally does not require surgery.

Is the second example more typical than the first? How frequently does my intuition mislead me? The Swedish study's radical consequence is that the customized, intuitive approach that underpins modern medicine is flawed—it generates more errors than it prevents. Studies conducted outside of medicine provide substantial evidence for this finding. Over the last four decades, cognitive psychologists have repeatedly demonstrated that a blind algorithmic method frequently outperforms human judgment when making predictions and diagnoses. In his classic 1954 treatise, Clinical Versus Statistical Prediction, psychologist Paul Meehl described a study of Illinois parolees that compared estimates given by prison psychiatrists that a convict would violate parole to estimates derived from a rudimentary formula that weighed factors such as age, number of previous offenses, and type of crime. Despite its crudeness, the model predicted the occurrence of parole violations much better than the psychiatrists did. In recent articles, Meehl and social scientists David Faust and Robyn Dawes reviewed over a hundred studies comparing computers or statistical formulas with human judgment in predicting everything from the likelihood of a company going bankrupt to the life expectancy of liver disease patients. In almost every situation, statistical thinking matched or outperformed human judgment. You could believe that humans and computers working together would make the best decisions. However, as the researchers point out, this claim makes little sense. It makes no difference if the viewpoints are in agreement. If they differ, research demonstrate that it's best to trust the computer's decision.

Physicians will almost certainly have to delegate some diagnostic judgments to machines. One network, PAPNET, has already found widespread use in the screening of digitized Pap smears—microscopic scrapings collected from a woman's cervix—for cancer or precancerous abnormalities, a task traditionally performed by a pathologist. Researchers have conducted over a thousand research on the application of neural networks in almost every aspect of medicine. Networks have been created to diagnose appendicitis, dementia, psychiatric problems, and sexually transmitted infections. Others can forecast success in cancer treatment, organ transplantation, and heart valve surgery. Systems have been developed to read chest X-rays, mammograms, and nuclear-medicine heart images.

In illness treatment, segments of the medical community have already begun to apply the Shouldice Hospital's lesson about the benefits of specialized, automated care. Regina Herzlinger, a Harvard Business School professor who coined the term "health-care focused factory" in her book Market-Driven Health Care, provides further examples, such as the Texas Heart Institute for cardiac surgery and Duke University's bone-marrow transplant center. Breast cancer patients appear to do best in specialist cancer treatment centers, where they have access to a cancer surgeon, an oncologist, a radiation therapist, a plastic surgeon, a social worker, a dietitian, and others who deal with breast cancer on a daily basis. Almost any hospital today has protocols and algorithms in place to treat at least a few common illnesses, such as asthma or a sudden stroke. The new artificial neural networks simply apply these lessons to the diagnosing process.

Nonetheless, resistance to this image of mechanized medicine will persist. Part of it could be a lack of foresight: doctors can be resistant to change the way things are done. Part of it, however, arises from valid concerns that, for all the technical virtuosity acquired, medicine loses something fundamental to machine. Modern care already lacks the human touch, and its technical attitude has alienated many of the individuals it claims to serve. Patients are already feeling like numbers far too often.

Chapter 3: When Doctors Make Mistakes

A few years back, at 2 a.m. on a crisp Friday in January, I was pulling a teenage knifing victim's abdomen open with sterile gloves and a gown when my pager rang. "Code Trauma, three minutes," the operating room nurse announced, reading aloud from my pager display. This indicated that another trauma patient would be transported to the hospital shortly, and as the surgical resident on duty for emergencies, I would be required to be present when the patient arrived. I stood back from the table and removed my gown. Two other surgeons were treating the knifing victim: Michael Ball, the attending (the staff surgeon in charge of the case), and David Hernandez, the top resident. Ordinarily, these two would have arrived to supervise and assist with the tragedy, but they were stuck here. Ball, a dry, analytical forty-two-year-old, glanced across at me as I walked toward the door. "If you run into any trouble, you call, and one of us will peel away," he told you.

The emergency room was one story up, and I arrived just as the emergency medical personnel dragged in a woman in her forties weighing over 200 pounds. She lay still on a hard orange plastic spinal board, eyes closed, complexion pale, and blood flowing from her nostrils. A nurse led the crew into Trauma Bay 1, an examination room designed like an operating room, complete with green tiles on the walls, monitoring gadgets, and space for portable X-ray equipment. We lifted her onto the bed and then got to work. One nurse started chopping off the woman's clothes. Another person took vital signs. A third placed a large-bore intravenous line in her right arm. A surgical intern placed a Foley catheter in her bladder. Samuel Johns, a thin guy in his fifties who resembled Ichabod Crane, was the emergency-medicine attendant. He was standing to one side, arms crossed, observing, which indicated that I could take charge.

Johns, the attending, wanted to perform the intubation. He grabbed a

Mac 3 laryngoscope, a standard but somewhat primitive-looking L-shaped metal equipment for prying open the mouth and throat, and inserted the shoehorn-like blade deep into her mouth and down to her larynx. Then he yanked the handle up toward the ceiling, removing her tongue, opening her mouth and throat, and revealing the voice chords, which look like fleshy tent flaps at the entrance to the trachea. The patient did not wince or gag; she was still unconscious. Johns removed everything from the patient's mouth before reattaching the bag mask. The oximeter's luminescent-green display briefly hovered at 60 before progressively rising to 97 percent. After a few minutes, he removed the mask and tried again to insert the tube. There was more blood, and there could have been some swelling as well; all of the prodding down the neck was probably not helping. The SAT plummeted to 60 percent. He pulled out and "bagged" her till she was back to 95 percent.

I listened to the patient's lungs again, and there was no collapse. "We need to get her tubed," Johns added. He removed the oxygen mask and tried again.

Somewhere in my mind, I must have been aware that her airway was closing due to voice cord swelling or blood. If it was and we couldn't get a tube in, she'd only have a chance of survival if we performed an emergency tracheotomy, which involves cutting a hole in her neck and placing a breathing tube through it. Another effort to intubate her may cause a spasm of the cords and an abrupt closure of the airway, which is exactly what occurred.

Johns stooped over the patient, attempting to place the tube into her vocal cords. When her seat sank back into the 60s, he paused and reapplied the mask. We stared at the display. The figures were not showing up. Her lips were still bluish. Johns pressed harder on the bellows to get more oxygen in.

People started scurrying everywhere. I tried not to panic and instead proceeded deliberately. I told the surgical intern to put on a sterile gown and gloves. I got an antiseptic solution off the shelf and poured an entire container of yellow-brown liquid onto the patient's neck. A nurse unwrapped the tracheostomy kit, which included sterile drapes and equipment. I put on a robe and a new pair of gloves while trying to figure out the steps. This is so straightforward, I tried to convince myself. The cricothyroid membrane is a thin, fibrous covering that sits at the base of the thyroid cartilage, also known as the Adam's apple. Cut through that and voilà! You are in the trachea. You insert a four-inch plastic tube shaped like a plumber's elbow joint, connect it to oxygen and a ventilator, and she's ready. So, that was the theory.

I draped some fabric over her torso, leaving the neck exposed. It appeared as thick as a tree. I felt for the boney protrusion of the thyroid cartilage. However, I couldn't feel anything through the layers of fat. I was overwhelmed by uncertainty—where should I cut? Should I make a horizontal or vertical incision? I despised myself for it. Surgeons never dither, whereas I did. I hit a vein while dissecting down with scissors and the intern holding the incision open with retractors. It didn't spill much blood, but there was plenty to cover the wound; I couldn't see anything. The intern placed his finger on the bleeder. I asked for suction. However, the suction was ineffective because the tube had become clogged with clot from the intubation efforts.

James O'Connor, a silver-haired, seen-it-all anesthesiologist, entered the room. Johns gave him a quick overview of the patient and allowed him take over ventilating her. Holding the scalpel in my right hand like a pen, I inserted the blade into the cut at the location where I suspected the thyroid cartilage was. I sliced through the underlying fat and tissue with small, sharp strokes, working blindly due to the blood and bad lighting, until I felt the blade scrape against the almost boney cartilage. I searched with the knife's tip, moving it along until I felt a gap. I pressed down strongly, hoping it was the cricothyroid membrane. I felt the tissue give unexpectedly and cut an inch-long opening. I took the tracheostomy tube and attempted to insert it, but something appeared to be preventing it. I twisted and spun it before finally jamming it in. Just then, Ball, the surgical attending, came. He rushed up to the bed and leaned in for a look. "Did you get it?" he inquired. I responded I thought so. The bag mask was attached to the open end of the trache tube. However, when the bellows were compressed, air simply gurgled out of the wound. Ball promptly donned gloves and a robe.

The patient's saturation had dropped so low that the oximeter could no longer detect it. Her heart rate gradually decreased, first to the 60s and then to the 40s. Then she lost her pulse completely. I placed my hands on her chest, locked my elbows, leaned over, and began performing chest compressions. Ball looked up from the patient and moved to face O'Connor. "I'm not going to get her an airway in time," he admitted. "You're going to have to try again from above." Essentially, he was acknowledging my failure. Attempting an oral intubation again was pointless—it was something to do instead than watching her die. I was struck and concentrated on performing chest compressions without glancing at anyone. I thought it was over.

We soon recognized the woman, whom I'll call Louise Williams; she was 34 years old and lived alone in a neighboring suburb. Her alcohol level upon arrival was three times the legal limit, which most likely contributed to her unconsciousness. She suffered a concussion, multiple lacerations, and substantial soft-tissue injury. However, X-rays and scans revealed no other injuries from the crash. That night, Ball and Hernandez transported her to the operating room to be fitted with a proper tracheostomy. When Ball came out and spoke with family members, he described the critical condition she was in when she arrived, the difficulties "we" had in gaining access to her airway, the disturbingly long period of time she had gone without oxygen, and his uncertainty about how much brain function she still had.

They listened without complaint; all they could do was wait.

Consider some more medical mishaps. In one case, a general surgeon left a huge metal device in a patient's belly, tearing through the intestine and bladder wall. In another case, a cancer surgeon performed a biopsy on the incorrect region of a woman's breast, delaying her cancer diagnosis by months. During a heart valve operation, a cardiac surgeon overlooked a minor but critical step, resulting in the patient's death. A general surgeon met a guy in the emergency room with abdominal pain and concluded he had a kidney stone; eighteen hours later, a CT scan revealed a rupturing abdominal aortic aneurysm, and the patient died shortly thereafter.

In 1991, the New England Journal of Medicine released a series of important studies from the Harvard Medical Practice Study, which examined over 30,000 hospital admissions in New York State. According to the study, approximately 4% of hospital patients experienced treatment-related problems that either delayed their hospital stay or led in disability or death, with two-thirds of such difficulties being caused by errors in care. One-fourth, or one percent, of admissions involved real negligence. It is estimated that up to 44,000 patients die each year as a result of medical blunders. Subsequent studies across the country have verified the prevalence of errors. In one short research of how physicians perform when patients experience a sudden cardiac arrest, 27 out of 30 clinicians made a mistake when using the defibrillator, such as charging it incorrectly or spending too much time figuring out how to use a specific model. According to a 1995 research, mistakes in drug administration—giving the wrong drug or the wrong amount, for example—occur approximately once per hospital stay, with the majority of cases being minor, but one percent of the time having catastrophic implications.

If errors were caused by a subset of dangerous doctors, malpractice cases would be concentrated in a small group, yet they follow a uniform, bell-shaped distribution. Most surgeons face at least one lawsuit during their careers. Studies on various sorts of errors have also revealed that repeat offenders are not the problem. Every year, almost everyone who cares for hospital patients makes severe mistakes, if not outright carelessness. As a result, doctors are rarely incensed when the press covers yet another medical horror story. They usually react differently: "That could be me." The crucial concern is not how to protect bad physicians from injuring patients, but how to keep excellent physicians from harming patients.

Medical malpractice lawsuits are a highly unsuccessful solution. Troyen Brennan, a Harvard law and public health expert, points out that previous research has continually failed to discover evidence that litigation reduces medical errors. Part of this could be due to the weapon's inaccurate nature. Brennan oversaw many investigations that followed up on individuals from the Harvard Medical Practice Study. He discovered that less than 2% of patients who received inadequate care ever filed a lawsuit. In contrast, only a small percentage of the patients who sued were indeed victims of improper care. And a patient's chances of winning a lawsuit were based primarily on how bad his or her outcome was, regardless of whether it was caused by disease or inevitable hazards of care.

Every Tuesday at five o'clock in my hospital, we gather in a tall, luxurious amphitheater adorned with oil pictures of the famous doctors whose exploits we are expected to emulate. All surgeons are expected to attend, from interns to the chairman of surgery; we are also joined by medical students on their surgical "rotation." An M&M can have nearly a hundred people. We check in, get a photocopied list of cases to be discussed, and take our seats. The first row is held by the most senior surgeons: terse, solemn men dressed in dark suits rather than scrubs, arranged like a panel of senators at a hearing. The chairman is a leonine figure in the seat closest to the plain wooden podium from which each case is delivered. The remaining surgical attendings are arranged in the next rows; they are often younger, and several are female. The chief inhabitants have donned long white coats and typically sit in the side rows. I join the crowd of other residents, all dressed in short white coats and green scrub pants, filling the back rows.

For each case, the chief resident from the relevant service—cardiac, vascular, trauma, etc.—collects the facts, takes the podium, and narrates the story. Here's a sample list of cases from a normal week (with some adjustments to protect confidentiality): a sixty-eight-year-old man who bled to death after heart valve surgery; a forty-seven-year-old woman who had to have a reoperation because of infection following an arterial bypass done in her left leg; a forty-four-year-old woman who had to have bile drained from her abdomen after gallbladder surgery; three patients who had to have reoperations for bleeding following surgery; a sixty-three-year-old man who had a cardiac arrest following heart bypass surgery; a sixty-six Ms. Williams' case, as well as my unsuccessful tracheostomy, were only one of many on this list. David Hernandez, the chief trauma resident, had studied the records and met with me and the others involved. When the moment came, he stepped up front and told what had occurred.

Hernandez is a towering, boisterous, good old boy who can tell a story, but M & M presentations are bloodless and concise. He said something like, "This was a 34-year-old female unrestrained driver in a high-speed rollover. The patient appeared to have stable vital signs at the scene, but was unresponsive and was transported by ambulance without being intubated. She arrived with a GCS of 7. The Glasgow Coma Scale (GCS) measures the severity of head injuries on a scale of three to fifteen. GCS 7 is in the comatose range. "Intubation attempts were unsuccessful in the ER, which may have contributed to airway closure. A cricothyroidotomy was attempted unsuccessfully."

These presentations can feel awkward. The chief residents, not the attending physicians, decide which cases to report. That keeps the attendings honest—no one can hide mistakes—but it puts the chief residents, who are, after all, subordinates, in a difficult situation. A certain amount of material is necessarily omitted in a successful M & M presentation, as does the use of many passive verbs. Nobody does a cricothyroidotomy incorrectly.

Ball went on to discuss the emergency attendant's failure to intubate Williams, as well as his own failure to be at her bedside when things spiraled out of hand. He emphasized the poor lighting and her extraordinarily broad neck, taking care not to make them seem like excuses but rather complicating facts. Some attendees shook their heads with compassion. A couple of them asked clarifying questions. Throughout, Ball's tone was impartial and detached. He had the air of a CNN news anchor describing riots in Kuala Lumpur.

Throughout the M & M, no one questioned why I hadn't sought for aid sooner or why I had the expertise and knowledge that Williams required. This is not to argue that my acts were considered appropriate. Rather, Ball's function in the hierarchy was to remedy my errors. The day after the disaster, Ball had stopped me in the hall and taken me aside. His voice was more wounded than angry as he recounted my specific shortcomings. First, he emphasized that in an emergency tracheostomy, it could have been wiser to make a vertical neck incision to keep me out of the blood arteries that go up and down—something I should have understood based on my reading. "I might have had a much easier time getting her an airway then," he said. Second, and even worse to him than ignorance, he couldn't comprehend why I hadn't called him when there were obvious indicators of airway trouble developing. I made no justifications. I promised to be better prepared in such situations and to seek assistance more quickly.

Even after Ball had left the fluorescent-lit hallway, I felt humiliation like a burning ulcer. This was not guilt; guilt is the emotion you experience after you have done something wrong. I felt ashamed: I was what was wrong. But I also knew that a surgeon could overreact to such feelings. It is one thing to recognize one's limitations. Being afflicted by self-doubt is something else entirely. One nationally recognized surgeon told me about an abdominal procedure in which he lost control of bleeding while removing what turned out to be a benign tumor, and the patient died. "It was a clean kill," he explained. He struggled to function after it. When he did operate, he grew hesitant and unsure. The case had a long-term impact on his performance.

In its own way, the M&M is an astonishingly smart and humane institution. Unlike the courts or the media, it accepts that punishment cannot discourage human mistake in most cases. The M & M considers preventing error to be mostly a matter of will—of remaining sufficiently aware and vigilant to foresee the various ways that things can go wrong and then attempting to head off each potential problem before it occurs. An error is not damnable, but it does bring some humiliation. In reality, the M&M ethos can appear incongruous. On the one hand, it fosters the distinctly American notion that error is intolerable. On the other hand, the M & M's very existence, as well as its presence on the weekly timetable, demonstrates an acceptance that mistakes are an unavoidable aspect of treatment.

But why do they occur so frequently? Lucian Leape, medicine's preeminent error specialist, notes that many other industries—whether manufacturing semiconductors or serving customers at the Ritz-Carlton—would simply not tolerate error rates as high as those in hospitals. The aviation sector has lowered the frequency of operational faults to one per hundred thousand flights, with the majority of those failures having no negative implications. The buzzword at General Electric these days is "Six Sigma," which means that the company's goal is to make product failures so rare that they are statistically more than six standard deviations away from being a matter of chance—roughly a one-in-a-million occurrence.

Of course, patients are far more difficult and idiosyncratic than airplanes, and medicine isn't just about supplying a fixed product or even a catalog of products; it could be more complex than almost any other sector of human endeavor. However, everything we've learned over the last two decades—from cognitive psychology, "human factors" engineering, and disaster studies like Three Mile Island and Bhopal—has given the same insights: not only do all humans make mistakes, but they do it repeatedly and in predictable, systematic ways. And solutions that do not account for these realities may end up aggravating rather than decreasing errors.

The M&M ignores all of this. As a result, many professionals regard it as a subpar strategy to assessing error and improving performance in medicine. It is not sufficient to inquire as to what a physician could or should have done differently so that he and others can learn from the experience in the future. The doctor is frequently the concluding actor in a series of events that set him or her up for failure. Error specialists feel that the process, rather than the individuals involved, deserves closer investigation and rectification. In a way, they seek to industrialize medicine. And they can already point to successes: the Shouldice Hospital's "focused factory" for hernia procedures, for example—and, far more widely, the entire specialty of anesthesiology, which has adopted their principles and achieved exceptional outcomes.

Obtaining open, honest reporting is critical. The Federal Aviation Administration has a systematic system for analyzing and reporting harmful aviation accidents, and its remarkable success in increasing airline safety is built on two foundations. Pilots who report an event within ten days are automatically exempt from penalties, and the reports are routed to a neutral, outside entity, NASA, which has no interest in utilizing the material against individual pilots. Jeffrey Cooper undoubtedly benefited from the fact that he was an engineer rather than a physician, as anesthesiologists saw him as a discreet, unthreatening researcher.

The end result was the first comprehensive scientific investigation into medical blunders. His meticulous investigation of three hundred and fifty-nine faults provides a unique perspective on the profession. Contrary to popular belief, occurrences occurred in the middle of anesthesia, when awareness fell, rather than at the beginning ("takeoff"). The most prevalent type of incident was faults in sustaining the patient's breathing, which were usually caused by an undetected disconnection or misconnection of the breathing tube, errors in controlling the airway, or errors in operating the anesthesia machine. Cooper also identified a number of contributing variables, including insufficient experience, unfamiliarity with equipment, poor team communication, hurry, inattention, and weariness.

Where errors could not be eliminated immediately, anesthesiologists began seeking for reliable ways to detect them sooner. Because the trachea and esophagus are so close together, it is practically unavoidable that an anesthesiologist will occasionally insert the breathing tube into the wrong pipe. Anesthesiologists had always checked for this with a stethoscope, listening for breath sounds in both lungs. Cooper, on the other hand, has discovered a remarkable number of catastrophes involving unreported esophageal intubations, such as the one that occurred with Pierce's friends' daughters. Something more effective was required. In fact, monitors capable of detecting this type of inaccuracy have been available for years, but due to their high cost, few anesthesiologists utilize them. One form of monitor might determine whether the tube was in the trachea by detecting carbon dioxide exhaled from the lungs. Another version, the pulse oximeter, monitored blood oxygen levels, offering an early signal that anything was amiss with the patient's respiratory system.

Prodded by Pierce and others, the anesthesiology organization established both types of monitors as an official norm for all patients getting general anesthesia. Today, anesthetic deaths caused by misconnecting the respiratory system or intubating the esophagus instead of the trachea are almost unknown. In a decade, the overall death rate fell to one in over two hundred thousand instances, or less than a sixteenth of what it had been.

Gaba, a physician with technical experience, was in charge of designing the Eagle Patient Simulator, an anesthesia simulation system. It is a life-size, computer-controlled mannequin capable of incredibly realistic behavior. It has a circulation, a heartbeat, and lungs that absorb oxygen and expel carbon dioxide. If you inject medications or give it inhaled anesthetics, it will identify the type and dosage, and its heart rate, blood pressure, and oxygen levels will adjust accordingly. The "patient" can be made to experience airway edema, hemorrhage, and cardiac problems. The mannequin is placed on an operating table in a simulation room that looks just like the real thing. Both residents and experienced attending physicians learn how to perform effectively in a variety of dangerous, and sometimes bizarre, scenarios, including an anesthesia machine malfunction, a power outage, a patient who goes into cardiac arrest during surgery, and even a cesarean-section patient whose airway closes and requires an emergency tracheostomy. Though anesthesiology has definitely led the way in examining and attempting to correct "systems" errors, there are hints of progress in other areas. The American Medical Association, for example, established the National Patient Safety Foundation in 1997 and appointed Cooper and Pierce to its board of directors. The organization is supporting research, hosting conferences, and working to set new standards for hospital drug-ordering systems that might significantly reduce medication errors—the most common sort of medical error.

The Northern New England Cardiovascular Disease Study Group, situated in Dartmouth, is another success story. Though the organization does not perform the type of in-depth research of catastrophes that Jeffrey Cooper pioneered, it has demonstrated what may be accomplished merely with statistical surveillance. This partnership, which includes six institutions, analyzes mortality and other negative events (such as wound infection, uncontrolled bleeding, and stroke) associated with heart surgery in order to determine the many risk factors. Its researchers discovered, for example, that there were relatively high fatality rates among patients who acquired anemia following bypass surgery, and that anemia occurred most frequently in tiny people. The anemia was induced by the fluid used to "prime" the heart-lung machine, which diluted a patient's blood. The smaller the patient (and his or her blood supply), the greater the effect. Members of the collaboration now have numerous viable answers to the challenge. Another study discovered that a group at one institution made mistakes in "handoffs"—for example, sending preoperative test data to those in the operation room. The study group solved the problem by creating a pilot checklist for all patients presenting to the OR. These initiatives increased standardization, lowering the fatality rate in those six institutions from 4% to 3% between 1991 and 1996. That meant two hundred and ninety-three less deaths. Despite its restricted focus and procedures, the Northern New England cardiac group remains an outlier; concrete data on how things go wrong is still scarce. There is a slew of evidence that latent errors and systemic factors may contribute to surgical errors, including a lack of standardized protocols, the surgeon's inexperience, the hospital's inexperience, inadequately designed technology and techniques, thin staffing, poor teamwork, time of day, the effects of managed care and corporate medicine, and so on.

It was a routine gallbladder procedure on a routine day: a mother in her forties lay on the operating table, her body draped in blue paper save for her round, antiseptically coated abdomen. The gallbladder is a floppy, finger-length sac of bile that sits beneath the liver, and gallstones, as this patient discovered, may cause agonizing discomfort. The agony would stop once we removed her gallbladder.

There are hazards associated with this operation, but they were much higher previously. merely a decade ago, surgeons had to make a six-inch abdominal incision, which kept patients in the hospital for about a week merely to recuperate from the wound. Today, we learned how to remove gallbladders using a micro camera and instruments inserted through tiny incisions. The procedure, which is frequently performed as day surgery, is known as laparoscopic cholecystectomy, or "lap chole." Every year, half a million Americans have their gallbladders removed in this manner; at my institution alone, we perform several hundred lap choles.

Removing the gallbladder is rather simple. You cut it from its stalk and blood supply, then take the rubbery sac out of the abdomen through an incision at the belly button. You let the carbon dioxide out of the belly, remove the ports, stitch up the little incisions, apply some Band-Aids, and you're done. However, there is one lurking danger: the gallbladder stalk is a branch of the liver's only channel for transferring bile to the intestines for fat breakdown. If you accidentally injure this primary bile duct, the bile accumulates and begins to kill the liver. Between 10 and 20 percent of patients who experience this will die. Those who survive generally have lifelong liver damage and may require a liver transplant. A textbook states: "Injuries to the main bile duct are nearly always the result of misadventure during operation and are therefore a serious reproach to the surgical profession." It is a true surgical error, and like any surgical team performing a lap chole, we were determined to avoid it.

I inserted the clip applier, a tool that squeezes V-shaped metal clips onto whatever you place in its jaws. I had my jaws around the duct and was about to fire when I noticed a small globule of fat on the screen. That wasn't very rare, but it just didn't look right. I tried to flick it aside with the tip of the clip applier, but instead of a small globule, a layer of thin, invisible tissue emerged, and underneath, we discovered that the duct had a bifurcation. My heart sank. Without that particular attention to detail, I would have severed the primary bile duct.

The story, however, does not have to end here, as cognitive psychologists and industrial error experts have proved. Given the results in anesthesiology, it's evident that focusing on the method rather than the individuals would result in huge gains. However, the industrial remedy has significant limits, despite its important emphasis on systems and structures. It would be fatal for us, as individual players, to abandon our trust in human perfection. The statistics may suggest that one day I will sever someone's major bile duct, but each time I undergo a gallbladder surgery, I think that with enough will and effort, I can overcome the chances. This is not simply professional vanity. It's an essential component of good medicine, even in highly "optimized" systems. Operations like that lap chole have taught me how quickly errors can occur, but they've also shown me that effort is important; vigilance and attention to the smallest details can save you. There are numerous reasons why it would be wrong to suspend my license or take me to court. These factors do not excuse me. Whatever its limitations, the M&M's uncompromising ethic of personal accountability for errors is a formidable virtue. Doctors will occasionally make mistakes, no matter what precautions are taken, and it is unreasonable to expect perfection. It is realistic to expect that we never stop aiming for it.

Chapter 4: Nine Thousand Surgeons

Conventions are a huge deal in medicine. My medical parents had been attending their conventions for thirty years, and I vaguely remembered how dense, big, and fascinating they appeared when they had taken me along as a child. As a resident, I had become accustomed to the operating schedule abruptly clearing out in mid-October, when the faculty surgeons went off to their annual convention en masse. But we residents would stay behind, together with a skeleton crew of unlucky attendings (generally the most junior ones), to handle the trauma patients and other random crises that continued to arrive. A lot of time was spent relaxing in the residents' lounge—a dull, musty area with flat brown carpeting, a moldering couch, a broken rowing machine, empty Coke cans, and two televisions—watching end-of-year baseball on the one working television and eating take-out Chinese.

Each year, a few senior citizens have been able to attend the gathering. And in my sixth year, I was told that I had progressed enough in training to be one of them. The hospital turned out to have a little fund that could pay for the trip. Within a few days, I had a plane ticket to Chicago, a hotel reservation at the Hyatt Regency, and an entry badge for the eighty-sixth annual Clinical Congress of Surgeons. It wasn't until I was at 27,000 feet in a Boeing 737 somewhere above New Hampshire, with my wife returning home for a week with sole custody of our three children, that I began to wonder what on earth people travel to these places for.

When we arrived, each of us was given a 388-page schedule of programs we could attend, ranging from a course on advanced image-guided breast biopsies on the first morning to a panel presentation on the sixth and final day titled "Office-Based Treatment of Ano-Rectal Disease—How Far Can We Go?". I eventually settled down with my book, carefully examining it page by page and highlighting everything that piqued my interest in blue ballpoint pen. This, I determined, was the place to find the new and better—the place to teach the practically perfect—and it felt almost a responsibility to attend as many of the events as possible. My book quickly became blue and covered in circles. On the first morning alone, I had over twenty informative-looking programs to pick from. I pondered attending a lecture on how to properly dissect a neck or a session on recent developments in handling gunshot wounds to the brain, but ultimately chose a panel debate on the best approach to repair groin hernias.

I arrived early, and the auditorium's fifteen hundred seats were already filled. Hernias were SRO. I found a spot to stand among the mob around the back wall. I could hardly see the lectern in front of me, but a massive television screen displayed close-ups of each of the speakers. Eleven surgeons, one after the other, took the platform to show Powerpoint presentations and argue about data.

In the afternoon, I visited the cinema. The organizers had set up three theaters, each seating three or four hundred people, to show reel after reel of actual activities throughout the day. I slipped into one gloomy chamber and was immediately captivated. I seen daring operations, sophisticated operations, and brilliantly simple operations. The first film I saw was from Memorial Sloan Kettering Cancer Center in Manhattan. It started with a close-up of a patient's open abdomen. The surgeon, unseen but for his gloved and bleeding hands, was undertaking an extremely difficult and risky operation: removing a malignancy from the tail of a patient's pancreatic. The tumor was deep, surrounded by loops of bowel, a latticework of blood arteries, the stomach, and the spleen. However, the surgeon made the extraction appear easy. He ripped at delicate veins and cut through tissue millimeters from vital organs. He showed us a few strategies for avoiding difficulties, and before we knew it, he had half of the pancreas on a platter.

The clinical sessions were scheduled until 10:30 p.m. each night, and they all seemed to follow the pattern of the first two I attended, ranging from the pedantic to the beautiful, the ordinary to the remarkable. If such programs were supposed to be the highlight of the meeting, it was sometimes difficult to discern. The convention quickly became clear that it was more of a trade event than an educational meeting. Advertisements for exciting new stuff you'd never heard of—a tissue-stapling gadget that staples without staples, a fiber-optic scope that allows you to view in three dimensions—ran night and day on my hotel room television and even on the shuttle bus to and from the convention center. Drug and medical device businesses invited people to complimentary dinners across town every night. And there were almost five thousand three hundred salespeople from twelve hundred organizations in attendance—more than one for every two surgeons.

Sometimes it was just chintzy, free items. Booths were handing out free golf balls, fountain pens, penlights, baseball caps, sticky pads, and candies, all stenciled with company logos and accompanied by a spiel and a pamphlet about some new technology being marketed. You may assume that six-figure surgeons would be immune to this type of petty bribery. But you would be mistaken. A medicine manufacturer hosted one of the busiest booths at the event, handing out durable white canvas bags with the name of one of its drugs painted in four-inch blue letters along the side. Doctors waited in line for the bags, even if it meant giving over their phone numbers and addresses in order to obtain something to carry all of the free items they were accumulating. (However, I overheard one physician complain that the pickings were not as good as in prior years. He had gotten Ray-Ban sunglasses once, he remarked.

After giving up on making it anywhere else that day, I noticed a gathering of about fifty surgeons swarming around a projection screen and a man wearing a suit and a headset microphone. I walked up to see what all the excitement was about, and what I saw was a live televised image of a patient having a big, prolapsed internal hemorrhoid removed in an operating room someplace in Pennsylvania. The company was demonstrating a new disposable device (cost: $250) that claimed to reduce the typical half-hour operation to less than five minutes. The emcee in the headset took questions from the audience, which he then posed to the surgeon as he worked a thousand miles away.

When the play ended, I observed a forlorn-looking pockfaced man in a rumpled brown suit sitting alone in a little booth. People rushed by him like minnows, with no one pausing to inspect his stuff. He had no television screens, brushed-steel displays, or free stenciled golf tees—just a computer-printed paper sign with no logo ("Scientia," it read) and several hundred vintage surgical volumes. Feeling sorry for him, I paused to explore and was astounded to see what he has to offer. He had, for example, Joseph Lister's original 1867 writings in which he described his groundbreaking antiseptic surgical approach. He owned the initial 1924 edition of the great surgeon William Halsted's collection of scholarly articles, as well as the original 1955 proceedings of the world's first organ transplant symposium. He had an 1899 catalogue of surgical instruments, a surgical textbook from two centuries ago, and a complete reproduction of Maimonides' medical work. He even obtained an 1863 logbook from a Union Army Civil War medic. There was a treasure trove of diamonds in his crates and shelves, and I spent the rest of the afternoon fascinated in them.

There was another area in the convention where you could be certain of seeing great things happening. The "Surgical Forums" took place in a cluster of small meeting rooms far from the major halls, where the movies were played, practical sessions were held, and merchandise was sold. Every day, researchers of all kinds met here to discuss their current projects. The disciplines included genetics, immunology, physics, and population statistics. The debates were lightly attended and generally went over my head: nowadays, it is impossible to understand even the most basic terms in all of the subjects under consideration. But while I sat there listening to the scientists discuss among themselves, I got a sense of where the edges of knowledge were, the reachable boundaries.

The researchers reported results from the first dozen patients. Each of the patients had reached the end stage of liver failure, at which point 90 percent of people die while waiting for a transplant. However, with the bioengineered liver, the researchers stated that all of them survived long enough to find a donor liver—in many cases for ten days or more, an unprecedented feat. Surprisingly, four patients in end-stage failure due to drug overdoses did not require a transplant. The bioengineered liver had sustained each for long enough for his or her own liver to heal and rebuild. Sitting in the crowd, I felt a rush of excitement as I realized what these doctors had done. And I began to wonder if it was similar to how Joseph Lister's colleagues at the Royal College of Surgeons felt when he first presented his antisepsis discoveries about a century and a half ago.

According to anthropologist Lawrence Cohen, conferences and conventions are more like carnivals than scholarly gatherings—"colossal events where academic proceedings are overshadowed by professional politics, ritual enactments of disciplinary boundaries, sexual liminality, tourism and trade, personal and national rivalries, the care and feeding of professional kinship, and the sheer enormity of discourse." This appears to be appropriate in surgical settings. It didn't take long to discover that some had come only to be seen, some to make a name for themselves, and still others for the sheer spectacle of it all. There were political contests (a new president and board of governors were elected), as well as private meetings. There were residency reunions. There were nights out at Spago, and there were almost certainly some love affairs.

Despite this, there was a sense that the appeal went beyond the carnival. You could see it, for example, on the bus. Every day, we surgeons traveled between the convention center and our lodgings in big tour buses. (They were similar to Greyhound's Atlantic City routes, but ours had drop-down mini-televisions advertising the "Surgical Zipper.") We were mostly strangers—I had never met anyone on those bus rides—but if you had seen us, it wouldn't have appeared that way. Consider the simple act of sitting. Normally, individuals boarding a bus, plane, or train distribute themselves like repelling magnets, maintaining a respectful, anonymous distance from one another and sharing seats only when necessary. However, as we boarded our busses, we decided to sit two-by-two despite the fact that other seats were empty. The social rules had been inverted, seemingly without anyone's knowledge. On any other bus in Chicago, a stranger sitting next to you would have made you feel almost physically threatened if three-quarters of the seats were empty. However, the guy who distinguished himself would have caused the most concern. You felt like you belonged to your tribe, even if you didn't know anyone. You felt compelled to say hi. It felt disrespectful not to do so.

This is, I believe, what public relations pros call networking. However, the term fails to capture the doctors' desperate want for interaction and belonging on those buses and during the convention. We may have all had fine practical reasons for coming here: new ideas, things to learn, gadgets to test, the pursuit of status, and a reprieve from the grind of never-ending duties. But, in the end, I realized there was something more vital and, in a way, poignant that drew us in.

Doctors live in an insular world of hemorrhages, lab tests, and patients being hacked open. We are currently the healthy few living amid the sick. And it is easy to get disconnected from the experiences and, at times, values of the rest of civilization. Ours is a world that our family do not understand. Athletes, soldiers, and professional musicians have all had similar experiences in some ways. Unlike them, we are not just separated, but also alone. Once residency is completed and you have settled in Sleepy Eye, the northern peninsula of Michigan, or, for that matter, Manhattan, the influx of patients and isolation of practice separate you from anyone who truly understands what it is like to cut a stomach cancer from a patient, lose her to pneumonia later, answer the family's accusing questions, or fight with insurers to get paid.

Chapter 5: When Good Doctors Go Bad

Hank Goodman was a retired orthopedic surgeon. He is fifty-six years old, stands six feet one, has thick, disheveled brown hair, and outsize hands that could easily pop a knee back into place. He is composed and assured, a man accustomed to repairing bones. Before his license was revoked, he was a well-known and popular surgeon. "He could do some of the best, most brilliant work around," one of his orthopedic colleagues told me. When other doctors required an orthopedist for relatives and friends, they turned to him. For over a decade, Goodman was one of the busiest surgeons in his state. But somewhere along the way, things began to go awry. He started to cut corners and became sloppy. Patients were injured, some severely. Colleagues who had once admired him became horrified. He was eventually stopped, but it took years.

When people talk about bad doctors, they usually refer to monsters. We read about doctors like Harold Shipman, a physician from the North of England who was convicted of murdering fifteen patients with deadly doses of opiates and is suspected of killing 300 in total. Or John Ronald Brown, a San Diego surgeon who, while working without a license, botched a series of sex-change procedures and severed the left leg of a perfectly healthy man, who later died of gangrene. Or James Burt, a prominent Ohio doctor who performed a weird, disfiguring operation including clitoral circumcision and vaginal "reshaping," known as the Surgery of Love, on hundreds of women, frequently after they had been anesthetized for earlier procedures.

One case started on a sweltering August day in 1991. Goodman was at the hospital, a tentacled, contemporary, floodlit complex with a towering red-brick building in the centre and many smaller buildings radiating out from it, all supplied by a vast network of outlying clinics and a nearby medical school. The operating rooms were located off a long corridor on the ground level of the main structure, with white-tiled, wide-open areas, patients arranged under a canopy of lights, and teams of blue-clad workers going about their business. Goodman completed an operation in one of these rooms, removed his gown, and went over to a wall phone to check his messages while waiting for the room to be cleaned. One came from his medical assistant's office, which was half a block away. He wanted to talk with Goodman about Mrs. D.

This explanation made it evident that the woman was suffering from a serious infection and needed to have her knee opened and drained as soon as possible. But Goodman was preoccupied, so he never considered the suggestion. He did not bring her into the hospital. He did not go to see her. He hadn't even had a colleague visit her. He advised her to take oral antibiotics. When the assistant expressed uncertainty, Goodman replied, "Ah, she's just a whiner."

A week later, the patient returned, and Goodman successfully drained her knee. Unfortunately, it was too late. The virus had destroyed the cartilage. Her whole joint was shattered. Later, she saw another orthopedist, but all he could do was solidify her knee to alleviate the continual discomfort of bone grinding against bone.

Every physician is capable of making a stupid, careless judgment like Goodman's, but in his latter years in practice, he did it often. In one example, he used the wrong-size screw to repair a patient's broken ankle and failed to discover that the screw had penetrated too far. When the patient complained about pain, Goodman refused to acknowledge that anything needed to be done. In a similar example, he inserted the incorrect size screw into a shattered elbow. The patient returned once the screw head had corroded through the skin. Goodman could have easily trimmed the screw to size, but he did not.

For the last few years of his career, Goodman was the defendant in a slew of malpractice actions, which he resolved as swiftly as possible. His bungled cases became a regular feature of his department's Morbidity and Mortality presentations. Goodman became a committed student, was accepted into an elite medical school, and plans to pursue a career in surgery after graduation. Following his military service as a general medical officer in the Air Force, he was admitted into one of the country's best orthopedic residency programs. Despite the long hours, he found the work to be quite rewarding. He was good at it. People came in with excruciatingly painful and crippling conditions—dislocated joints, fractured hips, limbs, and spines—and he repaired them. "Those were the four best years of my life," he told me. He then pursued specialist training in hand surgery, and when he finished in 1978, he had a diverse range of job opportunities. He ended up returning to the Northwest, where he spent the following fifteen years.

Things began to alter around 1990. With his skill and experience, Goodman knew better than most what needed to be done for Mrs. D, the man with the broken hip, and many other patients, but he didn't do it. What happened? All he could tell me was that everything seemed wrong during the last few years. He used to like being in the operation room and helping people. After a while, it appeared like all he cared about was getting through all of his patients as soon as possible. His professional identity made him unwilling to turn people away. (He was, after all, the one who never said no.) Whatever the reason, his caseload had clearly gotten onerous. He'd been working 80, 90, or 100 hours per week for well over a decade. He had a wife and three children, all of whom are now adults, although he rarely saw them. His calendar was crowded, and he needed to be as efficient as possible to get everything done. He'd start with, say, a total hip replacement at 7:30 a.m. and aim to finish in about two hours. Then he'd take off his gown, tear through the papers, and, as the room was being cleaned, march out the main tower doors, into the sun, snow, or rain, and across to the outpatient surgery facility, which was half a block away. He'd have another patient waiting on the table—a basic case like a knee arthroscopy or a carpal tunnel release. Near the end, he'd direct a nurse to call ahead and have the next patient carried into the OR in the main tower. He'd close the skin on the second case and then rush back for the third. He moved back and forth all day. Despite his efforts to keep up, unforeseen complications arose—a delay in preparing a room, a new patient in the emergency room, an unexpected difficulty during a surgery. He eventually found the snags excruciating. That's probably when things got dangerous. Medicine demands the willpower to accept what comes: your calendar may be jam-packed, the hour late, and your child waiting for you to pick him up from swimming practice; yet, if a problem emerges, you must do what is necessary. Goodman repeatedly failed to do so.

There is an official line on how the medical profession is supposed to deal with these physicians: colleagues are expected to band together immediately to remove them from practice and report them to the medical-licensing authorities, who are then supposed to discipline or expel them from the profession. It almost never happens that way. For no close-knit community can function in that manner.

Marilynn Rosenthal, a sociologist at the University of Michigan, investigated how medical communities in the United States, Great Britain, and Sweden deal with problematic physicians. She has gathered data on what transpired in over 200 unique cases, ranging from a family physician with a barbiturate addiction to a 53-year-old heart surgeon who continued to operate despite severe cerebral impairment from stroke. And almost wherever she glanced, she saw the same thing. It took months, if not years, for colleagues to take effective action against a terrible doctor, no matter how dangerous his or her conduct was.

People have referred to this as a conspiracy of silence, but Rosenthal discovered a glaring absence of plotting. In the communities she has studied, the dominating reaction has been uncertainty, denial, and hesitant, feckless intervention—similar to a family that refuses to admit that grandma's driver's license needs to be revoked. For starters, not all problems are obvious: colleagues may assume that Dr. So-and-So drinks too much or has gotten "too old," but certainty on such matters might be difficult to obtain for a long time. Furthermore, even when problems are clear, colleagues frequently find themselves unwilling to take immediate action.

There are both noble and despicable motivations for this. The shameful explanation is that doing nothing is simple. Colleagues must put in a tremendous amount of effort and confidence to compile the evidence and votes required to suspend another doctor's practicing privileges. The honorable reason, and most likely the primary reason, is because no one truly cares about it. When a skilled, nice, and normally diligent colleague, whom you've known and worked with for years, begins taking Percodans or becomes obsessed with personal issues and neglects proper patient care, you want to help, not destroy the doctor's career. However, there are no simple solutions. In private practice, there are no sabbaticals or leaves of absence; only disciplinary proceedings and public reports of wrongdoing. As a result, when people attempt to help, they do so quietly and privately. Their intentions are good, but the results are typically not.

For a long time, Hank Goodman's coworkers attempted to assist him. They had suspicions about 1990. There was discussion of odd rulings, dubious outcomes, and an increasing number of lawsuits. People felt increasingly compelled to intervene.

As is frequently the case, the people in the best position to observe how dangerous Goodman had become were also in the weakest position to intervene: junior physicians, nurses, and ancillary staff. In such cases, the support team will frequently take precautions to protect patients. Nurses find themselves quietly referring patients to other providers. Receptionists are suddenly having problems locating openings in a doctor's schedule. Senior surgical residents observe junior-level operations to ensure that a particular surgeon does not cause injury.

One of Goodman's physician assistants attempted to take on the protecting role. When he first started working with Goodman—setting fractures, tracking patients' progress, and aiding in the operating room—he admired the man. However, he observed when Goodman got inconsistent. "He'd run through forty patients in a day and not spend five minutes with them," the assistant explained. To avoid complications at the clinic, he stayed after hours to double-check Goodman's judgments. "I was constantly following up with patients and changing what he did for them." In the operation room, he attempted to offer friendly suggestions. "Is that screw too long?" he would inquire. "Does the alignment on that hip look right?" Nonetheless, there were mistakes and "a lot of unnecessary surgery," he admitted. When possible, he directed patients away from Goodman—"though without actually coming out and saying, 'I think he's crazy.'"

Matters can drift in this direction for an inconceivably long time. However, when someone has depleted all reservoirs of goodwill—when the Terribly Quiet Chats are plainly going nowhere and there appears to be no end to the behind-the-scenes work colleagues must do—the mood can shift quickly. The tiniest detail might trigger extreme action. Goodman began skipping the mandated weekly Morbidity and Mortality conferences in late 1993. People were still hesitant to judge him, no matter how bad his patient care was—he had become one of the hospital's most often sued doctors. When Goodman stopped going to M&Ms, his coworkers finally had a tangible violation to accuse him of.

Several individuals cautioned him, with growing vehemence, that he would be in big trouble if he didn't start turning up at M & Ms. "But he ignored them all," one of his colleagues told me. Following a year of this, the hospital board placed him on probation. Throughout it all, he was operating on more people, resulting in additional difficulties. Another year went by. Soon after Labor Day in 1995, the board and its lawyer sat him down at the end of a long conference table and informed him that they were suspending his operating privileges and submitting his actions to the state medical board for inquiry. He got fired.

Goodman had never told his family about his problems, and he hadn't told them he'd lost his work. He dressed in a suit and tie and went to his office every morning for weeks, as if nothing had changed. He visited the last of his scheduled patients and referred those who required surgery to others. Within a month, his practice was no longer viable. His wife realized something was wrong, and when she pressed him, he finally revealed everything. She was stunned and terrified; she felt like he was a stranger, an impostor. After that, he stayed at home in bed. He didn't speak to anyone for days at a time.

He had a .44 Magnum rifle in his basement den to protect himself from bears after purchasing it for a fishing trip to Alaska. He discovered the ammunition for the rifle and considered suicide. He knew how to ensure his death was swift. He was after all a surgeon.

In 1998, while skimming through the lengthy lecture schedule at a medical conference near Palm Springs, I came upon an interesting presentation: "Two Hundred Physicians Reported for Disruptive Behavior," by Kent Neff, M.D. The seminar was place in a tiny classroom located apart from the main lecture hall. At most, a few dozen people came. Neff was fiftyish, trim, silver-haired, and earnest, and he turned out to have what must be the most secretive specialism in medicine: he was a psychiatrist who specialized in doctors and other professionals with major behavioral issues. He told us that in 1994, he oversaw a tiny initiative that assisted hospitals and medical groups in dealing with troublesome doctors. They soon began sending him doctors from all over. He'd seen over 250 cases thus far, a remarkable quantity of experience, and he sifted over the data he'd gathered like a CDC scientist examining a tuberculosis outbreak.

His findings were unsurprising. Doctors were often not recognized as hazardous until they had caused significant damage. They were rarely given a full assessment for addiction, mental disease, or other common ailments. And, when problems were discovered, the follow-up was poor. What interested me was Neff's alone, quixotic attempt to address this issue—he had no grants or aid from any entities.

Several months after the speech, I flew to Minneapolis to watch Neff in action. His program was held at Abbott Northwestern Hospital, near the city's Powderhorn district. When I arrived, I was escorted to the fifth floor of a brick building hidden away to one side of the main hospital complex. There, I discovered a long, barely lighted hallway with closed, unmarked doors on both sides and beige, low-pile carpeting. It didn't look like a hospital. A block-lettered sign said "Professional Assessment Program." Neff, dressed in a tweed jacket and metal-rimmed spectacles, walked out one of the doors and showed me around.

Each Sunday night, the physicians arrived with luggage in hand. They checked in down the hall and were shown to dormitory-style rooms where they would spend four days and four nights. During the time I attended, there were three doctor-patients staying. They were free to come and go as they wanted, Neff assured me. But I knew they weren't quite free. In most cases, their hospitals had paid the program's $7,000 fee and informed the doctors that if they wanted to keep their practices, they needed to relocate to Minneapolis.

The most startling part of the program, in my opinion, was that Neff had successfully persuaded medical groups to send the doctors. He had accomplished this, it appeared, merely by volunteering to assist.

Despite their hesitation, hospitals and clinics expressed a strong desire for Neff's support. And they were not the only ones. Before long, airlines began sending him pilots. Courts assigned him judges. Companies sent him CEOs.

A small portion of what Neff did was simply meddle. He was like one of those physicians you see for a coughing child, and then they tell you how to live your life. He'd heed the physicians' advice, but he wasn't afraid to tell organizations when they'd let a problem fester too long. He says that certain types of behavior—what he refers to as "behavioral sentinel events"—should signal people that something is badly wrong with someone. A surgeon, for example, may toss scalpels in the operating room, while a pilot may become enraged in the middle of the flight. Nonetheless, such incidents are routinely ignored. "He's a fine doctor," people would say, "but sometimes he has his moments."

On the last day, Neff assembled his team around a conference table in a drab little room to make their determinations. Meanwhile, the physicians waited in their rooms. The staff members spent about an hour reviewing the data in each case. Then, as a team, they made three separate decisions. First, they arrived at a diagnosis. Most doctors turned out to have a psychiatric illness—depression, bipolar disorder, drug or alcohol addiction, even outright psychosis. Almost without exception, the condition had never been diagnosed or treated. Others were simply struggling with stress, divorce, grief, illness, or the like. Next, the team decided whether the doctor was fit to return to practice. Neff showed me some typical reports. The judgment was always clear, unequivocal: "Due to his alcoholism, Dr. X cannot practice with reasonable skill and safety at this time." Last, they spelled out specific recommendations for the doctor to follow. For some doctors deemed fit to return to practice, they recommended certain precautions: ongoing random drug testing, formal monitoring by designated colleagues, special restrictions on the doctor's practice. For those found unfit, Neff and his team typically specified a minimum period of time away from their practice, a detailed course of treatment, and explicit procedures for reevaluation. At the end of the deliberations, Neff met in his office with each doctor and described the final report that would be sent to his hospital or clinic. "People are usually surprised," Neff told me. "Ninety percent find our recommendations more stringent than what they were expecting."

Yet his program was shuttered a few months after my visit. Although it had attracted wide interest across the country and had grown rapidly, the Professional Assessment Program had struggled financially, never quite paying its own way. In the end, Neff was unable to persuade Abbott Northwestern Hospital to continue to subsidize it. He was, when we last spoke, seeking support to set up elsewhere.

Kent Neff saved Hank Goodman's life, and possibly his career as well. After considering suicide in mid-December 1995, Goodman called Neff's office. Goodman's lawyer had heard about the program and given him the phone number. Neff instructed him to come immediately away. Goodman traveled the next day. They met for an hour, and Goodman recalls feeling relieved at the conclusion. Neff was straightforward and collegial, telling him that he could help him and that his life was not finished. Goodman believed him.

He enrolled in the program the next week and paid for it himself. It was a challenging, often combative four days. He wasn't ready to own his mistakes or accept everything Neff's team discovered. The major diagnosis was long-term depression. Their judgment was characteristically blunt: The doctor, they concluded, "is unable to practice safely now because of his major depression and will be unable to practise for an indefinite period of time." According to the study, with sufficient and sustained therapy, "we would expect that he has the potential for a full return to practice." The specific diagnostic labels they assigned him are probably less essential than the intervention itself: telling him, with institutional authority, that something was wrong with him, that he should not practice, and that he might be able to do so again sometime.

We are all in the hands of fallible humans, no matter what we do. The truth is difficult to face. But it is unavoidable. Every doctor has things he or she should know but has yet to learn, judgmental capacities that will fail, and character strengths that can break. Was I stronger than he was now? More reliable? More conscientious? As attentive and cautious about my limitations? I wanted to think so—and maybe I had to think so in order to do what I do on a daily basis. But I couldn't know that. Neither could anyone else.

Goodman and I went out for a supper in town followed by a drive. When I arrived at his former hospital, which was shiny and contemporary, I asked him if I might look around. He didn't have to come, I explained. He had only been inside the building two or three times in the past four years. After a brief delay, he decided to accompany me. We entered through the sliding automatic doors and down a pristine white hallway. A bright voice burst out, and I could see he regretted coming in. He made an uncomfortable remark about all of the fishing he was going to do. We began walking away. Then he paused and spoke to her again. "I'll be back," he stated.

Part 2; Mystery

Chapter 6; Full Moon Friday the Thirteenth

Jack Nicklaus refused to play a round of golf without three pence in his pocket. Michael Jordan was always required to wear University of North Carolina boxer shorts under his Chicago Bulls uniform. And Duke Ellington would never do a gig, or allow his band members to perform one, while wearing anything yellow. Superstitions appear to be almost de rigueur among those who must perform for a living. Baseball players, for example, are famously superstitious. Wade Boggs, the Boston Red Sox's former standout third baseman, was known for eating chicken before every game. Tommy Lasorda, on the other hand, always ate linguine—with red clam sauce if his side was facing a right-handed pitcher and white if up against a lefty. Even amid this crowd, Turk Wendell, the pitcher for the New York Mets, appears strange. For luck during games, he used to wear an animal-fang necklace, refuse to wear socks, never stand on the foul line, and brush his teeth in between innings. When he signed his contract for the 1999 season, he demanded that his pay be $1,200,000.99.

So it struck me as odd when, one afternoon, as I and my fellow surgical residents sat around a table dividing up the next month's schedule of nights on emergency room duty, no one offered to take Friday the thirteenth. We were taking turns making choices, and for the first several rounds, everything seemed normal. We left all of the Fridays alone because weekend nights were not popular. But when the remaining evenings shrank to a few, it became clear that that one Friday was being deliberately avoided. Come on, I thought, this is ludicrous. So, when my turn came up again, I signed up for duty that night. "Rest up," one resident said. "You're going to be in for a busy night." I laughed and disregarded the idea. Looking at my calendar a few days later, I realised that the moon will likewise be full on

Friday night. Then someone noted that a lunar eclipse will also occur around that time. And for a little minute, I felt my confidence slipping. Perhaps I would have a bad night, I began to think. But as a sober and well-trained doctor, I refused to submit to such notions. Surely, I reasoned, the evidence is against such absurdity. After that, I went to the library to double-check.

Still, I told myself, you can't get much out of one study of a Friday the 13th in one town. Random fluctuation could easily have explained the increase in crashes. To be convinced, you'd need to observe consistently terrible results across multiple research. And that has yet to be demonstrated.

The Texas-sharpshooter fallacy refers to the tendency to see patterns that do not exist. Like a Texas sniper shooting at the side of a barn and then drawing a bull's-eye around the bullet holes, we tend to notice unexpected events first—four negative things happening on the same day, for example—and then construct a pattern around them. It appears that we could have feared Thursday the thirteenth or Friday the fifth just as much as Friday the thirteenth. Nonetheless, fear of Friday the thirteenth is common. According to surveys, Donald Dossey, a North Carolina behavioural scientist, estimates that between seventeen million and twenty-one million Americans experience mild to severe anxiety or adjust their activities due to paraskevidekatriaphobia (which is Greek for "fear of Friday the thirteenth"). They undertake rituals before leaving the house, call in sick to work, or postpone flights or large purchases, causing firms to lose $750 million each year.

Other types of madness appear to be unaffected by the moon. Researchers examined logs of calls to police stations, consultations with psychiatrists, killings, and other evidence of our daily weight of madness—including, I observed, emergency room visits. They discovered no continuous link with the moon. This reassured me, and I was finally able to leave the library confident that neither the full moon nor the unlucky date posed a threat to my night on call. A few weeks later, the scheduled evening arrived. I came into the ER at 6 p.m. sharp to take over for the daytime resident. To my dismay, he was already overloaded with patients for me to see. Then, just as I was getting caught up, a new catastrophe struck—a pallid and bloodied twenty-eight-year-old knocked unconscious in a high-speed head-on collision. Police and EMS say he was stalking his girlfriend with a gun. When cops came, he escaped in his car, leading them on a chase that resulted in the massive disaster.

Chapter 7: The Pain Perplex

Rowland Scott Quinlan's pain has a story, and it began with an accident when he was fifty-six years old. Quinlan, a Boston architect and passionate sailor with a shock of white hair and a preference for bow ties and Dutch cigarillos, led a booming Beacon Street firm in his name and developed structures such as the University of Massachusetts Medical School. Then, in March 1988, he fell over a board on the construction site of one of his assignments, a pavilion at Franklin Park Zoo. His back was good, but he dislocated and fractured his left shoulder, necessitating several surgeries. In the fall, he returned to his drafting table and was struck with a back spasm like a writhing serpent. The attacks continued, and while he initially tried to ignore them, they quickly became terrible. More than once, when standing with a client, his back pain suddenly flared up, and it was all he could do not to cry out as the client seized him and led him to a seat or the floor. He was sitting at a restaurant with a coworker when he was overtaken with anguish to the point of vomiting. Soon, he couldn't work more than two or three hours each day and had to hand over the firm to his partners.

When doctors see a patient with chronic pain who has no medical evidence to explain it—which is extremely common—they are dismissive. We believe the world is decipherable and logical, and that problems may be seen, felt, or measured with a machine. So we're likely to conclude that Quinlan's suffering is all in his head: not a physical ache, but a different, somehow less genuine, "mental" pain. In fact, Quinlan's orthopedist suggested that he consult both a psychiatrist and a physical therapist. When I visited Quinlan at his house in a seaside hamlet outside Boston, I found him sitting at his normal spot: a kitchen work table facing a wall-length window with a view of a little garden. Blueprints for incomplete constructions were curled up in rolls on the table. A telephone headset rested on one side. A dozen different types of drawing pens, as well as miniature rulers and a protractor, were stored in a holder. He scowled as he stood to greet me.

However, there are aspects of the agony that puzzle her and make her wonder if it is all in his brain. She sees that when he is upset or irritated, the pain worsens, yet when he is in a good mood or preoccupied, the discomfort subsides. He experiences spells of depression, which seem to trigger horrible spasms regardless of what he is doing physically. She, like his doctors, is perplexed as to how a pain can be so incapacitating yet having no discernible medical cause. What about the circumstances that trigger an attack—a mood, an idea, or nothing at all? These characteristics strike her as strange, requiring explanation. But the terrible truth is that Roland Scott Quinlan is not unique. His scenario is entirely common for chronic pain patients.

Dr. Edgar Ross, a forty-year-old anesthesiologist, directs the chronic-pain treatment centre at Brigham and Women's Hospital in Boston, where Quinlan is being treated. Dr. Ross sees patients with many types of pain, including back pain, neck pain, arthritis, total-body pain, neuropathic pain, AIDS-related pain, pelvic pain, chronic headaches, cancer pain, and phantom-limb pain. Frequently, they have already seen numerous doctors and attempted multiple therapy, including surgery, with no success. Ross escorted me to his office. He is soft-spoken and unhurried, with a calm disposition that is ideal for his job. Quinlan told me that this is the most common type of problem he encounters. Chronic back pain is now the second leading cause of lost work time, after only the common cold, and accounting for around 40% of workers' compensation payouts. In fact, this country is seeing a near pandemic of back pain, and no one knows why. Conventionally, we think of it as a mechanical condition caused by misdirected tension on the spine. As a result, we've had almost sixty years of workplace programs, and there are even "back schools," which teach the "correct way to lift," among other things.

Despite the fact that the number of persons engaged in manual labour has continuously reduced, more people than ever before suffer from chronic back pain.

More than three centuries ago, Rene Descartes developed the explanation for pain that has dominated much of medical history. Descartes claimed that pain is a purely physical phenomenon, in which tissue injury stimulates certain nerves, which send an impulse to the brain, allowing the mind to experience pain. He compared the occurrence to tugging a rope to ring a bell in the brain. It is difficult to emphasise how pervasive this account has grown. Pain research in the twentieth century has been primarily focused on the identification and study of pain-specific nerve fibres (now known as A-delta and C fibres) and pathways. In everyday medicine, clinicians view pain in Cartesian terms—as a physical process and an indication of tissue harm. We look for a ruptured disk, a fracture, an infection, or a tumour and try to treat the problem.

The shortcomings of this mechanical theory, however, have been known for some time. Lieutenant Colonel Henry K. Beecher, for example, conducted a seminal study of troops who had suffered catastrophic battlefield injuries during WWII. According to the Cartesian approach, the degree of harm should determine the degree of pain, much like a dial controlling volume. However, 58 percent of the men—men with complicated fractures, gunshot wounds, and torn limbs—reported only minor or no pain at all. Only 27% of the guys reported feeling enough pain to request pain medicine, despite the fact that comparable wounds are routinely treated with opiates in civilians. Clearly, something was going on in their minds—Beecher believed they were pleased to have escaped alive from the battlefield—that contradicted the signals conveyed by their injuries. Pain was being understood as significantly more nuanced than a one-way communication from injury to "ouch."

In 1965, Ronald Melzack, a Canadian psychologist, and Patrick

Wall, a British physiologist, proposed replacing the Cartesian model with the Gate-Control Theory of Pain. Melzack and Wall proposed that before pain signals reach the brain, they must pass through a gating mechanism in the spinal cord that can ratchet them up or down. In other situations, this hypothetical barrier could simply prevent pain impulses from reaching the brain. Researchers quickly discovered a pain gate in the dorsal horn of the spinal cord. The hypothesis solved simple puzzles like why stroking a painful foot makes it feel better. (Rubbing transmits signals to the dorsal horn, which closes the gate on neighbouring pain impulses.)

The findings were remarkable. On average, female students reported pain at sixteen seconds and removed their hands from the icy water at thirty-seven seconds. Female dancers took nearly three times as long on both counts. Men in both groups showed a higher threshold and tolerance for pain—as expected, given that studies reveal women to be more sensitive to pain than men, except during the last few weeks of pregnancy—but the gap between male dancers and male nondancers was virtually equal. What explains the difference? It's most likely related to the psyche of ballet dancers, who are known for their self-discipline, physical fitness, and competitiveness, as well as a high percentage of chronic injuries. Their driven personality and competitive culture clearly injure them to pain, which is why they can perform despite sprains and stress fractures, and why half of all dancers sustain long-term injuries. (Like most non-dancing males, I began to feel pain after about 25 seconds, but I had no issue keeping my hand in for the entire hundred and twenty seconds. I'll let others comment on what this means for the submissiveness instilled in surgical residents.

On a spring day in 1994, Dr. Frederick Lenz, a neurosurgeon at Johns Hopkins Hospital, saw a patient with significant hand tremors. The patient, whose I'll call Mark Taylor, was just 36 years old, but his hands had become so shaky over the years that even the most basic actions, such as writing, buttoning his shirt, sipping from a glass, or typing on his keyboard at his work as a purchasing agent, became impossibly difficult. Medications failed, and he lost jobs on multiple occasions as a result of his issues. Desperate to return to normal life, he agreed to a delicate procedure: brain surgery to remove cells in the thalamus, a tiny region known to contribute to excessive hand stimulation.

Taylor, on the other hand, had been suffering from a severe panic disorder for the previous seventeen years. At least once a week, while working at his computer terminal or nursing a child in the kitchen, he would have acute chest pains, as if he were suffering a heart attack. His heart would pound, his ears would ring, he'd get short of breath, and he'd have a strong want to go. Nonetheless, the psychologist Lenz consulted told him that the illness was unlikely to impede the procedure.

Initially, Lenz claims, everything went as expected. He injected a local anaesthetic—the procedure is performed while the patient is awake—and buried a small incision in Taylor's skull. Then he carefully inserted a long, thin electrical probe deep within, right into the thalamus. Lenz talked to Taylor the entire time, urging him to stick out his tongue, move a hand, or perform any of a dozen other activities that indicated he was fine. The hazard of this form of surgery is that it may damage the incorrect cells: the thalamic cells involved in tremor are only a fraction of a millimetre away from cells required for sensation and motor activity. So, before cauterising with a second, larger probe, the surgeon needed to locate the appropriate cells by stimulating them with a moderate electric pulse. The probe was in a section of Taylor's thalamus called Site 19, which Lenz shocked with low voltage. He had been here a thousand times previously, and he told me that zapping the place usually causes individuals to feel a prickle in their forearm. This is exactly how Taylor felt. Lenz then zapped an adjacent location he called Site 23, which often elicits a modest and relatively common sensation in the chest. This time, however, Taylor felt an unexpectedly far more severe pain—in fact, the precise chest pain of his panic attacks, complete with suffocation and an overwhelming sensation of doom. He cried out and nearly jumped off the table. When Lenz halted the stimulation, the sensation went away, and Taylor was quickly calm again. Puzzled, Lenz zapped Site 23 again, only to discover that the result was the same. He paused, apologised to Taylor for the discomfort, and then proceeded to pinpoint and cauterise the cells regulating his tremor. The procedure was successful.

Even as Lenz finished the treatment, his mind raced. He had only seen an impact like this once before. It occurred in a sixty-nine-year-old woman with a lengthy history of difficult-to-manage anginal discomfort that occurred not only during severe activity, but also during light physical exertion that would not normally stress her heart rate. Performing a similar surgery on her, Lenz discovered that stimulating the small area of her brain that ordinarily causes minor chest tingling had instead, like with Taylor, resulted in more acute and familiar chest pain—a sensation she characterised as "deep, frightful, squeezing." The consequences may have easily been overlooked, but Lenz had spent years researching pain and knew he had seen an important and telling effect. As he later stated in a research published in the journal Nature Medicine, the response in these two individuals was much out of proportion to the stimulation. What most people experience as a tingling sensation was anguish for them. Areas of the brain that control everyday feelings looked to have grown excessively sensitive—set to activate in response to completely harmless stimuli. In the woman's instance, her chest pain began as an indication of her heart condition but now appeared in settings that did not suggest an approaching heart attack. Even more curiously, Taylor's suffering began with his panic disorder, which is thought to be a psychiatric ailment. Lenz's findings show that, in reality, all pain is "in the head"—and that, in some cases, such as with Mark Taylor or Roland Scott Quinlan, no physical harm is required for the pain system to malfunction.

This is the most recent theory of pain. Its major proponent is Melzack, who abandoned Gate-Control Theory in the late 1980s and began telling sceptical audiences to change their understanding of pain once more. Given the data, he believes we should abandon the notion that pain or any other feeling is a passive "felt" input in the brain. Yes, injury causes nerve signals to go through a spinal-cord gate, but the pain perception is generated by the brain, which can do so even when no external stimuli are present. Melzack claims that even if a mad scientist reduced you to nothing more than a brain in a jar, you could still feel pain and have a full spectrum of sensory experience.

Suddenly, a basic toe-stub does not appear so simple. According to this viewpoint, the signal from the toe must still pass via the spinal cord gate before joining a slew of other signals in the brain, including those from memories, anticipation, mood, and diversions. Together, they may activate a neuro module that causes toe discomfort. In some persons, however, the tactile stimulus may be cancelled out, and the stubbed toe is barely noticeable. So yet, nothing unusual has happened. But now we may imagine—and this is the most radical aspect of Melzack's ideas—that the same neuro module can activate, causing actual toe pain, even if no toes have been stubbed. The neuro module, like Site 23 in Mark Taylor's brain, might be programmed to function as a hair trigger. Then almost anything could trigger it: a touch, a stab of terror, a sudden frustration, or a simple remembrance.

The new pain psychology hypothesis has, almost paradoxically, helped guide pain medication. For pharmacologists, the Holy Grail of chronic pain therapy is a tablet that is more effective than morphine but does not have the same side effects, such as dependence, drowsiness, and motor impairment. If an overactive neural system is the problem, what is required is a medication to calm it down. That is why, in what may have appeared unusual a decade ago, pain experts are increasingly prescribing anti-epileptic medications such as carbamazepine and gabapentin to their most difficult-to-treat patients. After all, that is what these medications do: they adjust brain cells to control their excitability. So yet, these types of medications work only for some people—Quinlan has been on gabapentin for more than six months with no effect—but drug companies are hard at work developing a new generation of similar "neuro-stabilising" substances.

At best, these medications offer only a partial remedy. The important issue for study is how to prevent the pain system in such patients from going crazy in the first place. People's stories of chronic pain generally begin with an injury. So, historically, we have attempted to prevent chronic pain by avoiding acute stresses. This concept sparked the development of an entire ergonomics sector. However, Ross's pain clinic and Lenz's operating table teach us that the causes of pain are not limited to the patients' muscles and bones. In fact, several types of chronic pain behave remarkably like social epidemics.

In the early 1980s, workers in Australia, particularly keyboard operators, experienced a sudden outbreak of severe arm discomfort, which doctors diagnosed as "repetitive strain injury," or RSI. This was not a moderate case of writer's cramp, but rather acute agony that began with modest discomfort while typing or performing other repetitive tasks and escalated to invalidism. The average period a person missed work was seventy-four days. As with persistent back pain, no consistent medical abnormalities or effective treatment could be detected, yet the arm discomfort spread like wildfire. It had barely existed before 1981, but by 1985, it had impacted a massive number of employees. In two Australian states, RSI crippled up to 30% of the workforce in particular industries, although pockets of workers remained mostly unaffected. Clusters formed even within the same organisation. At Telecom Australia, for example, the prevalence of RSI among telephone operators in a single city varied greatly across departments. Investigators were also unable to uncover a link between RSI and the workers' physical situations, such as the repetitive nature of their occupations or the ergonomics of their equipment. The outbreak then came to an abrupt end. By 1987, it had essentially ended. In the late 1990s, Australian researchers complained that there weren't enough RSI patients to investigate.

Chronic back pain has been with us for so long that it is difficult conceptually—and even politically—to take a step back and understand its social aetiology, let alone figure out how cultural variables disrupt an individual's pain system. The Australian pain pandemic reveals the potency of those elements to produce true, crippling pain on a national scale, but our understanding of their causes and how to mitigate them is limited. A variety of studies have shown that social-support networks, such as a good marriage and a fulfilling job, can protect against crippling back pain. We know, statistically speaking, that being assigned certain diagnostic designations and receiving disability pay (and hence some form of official acknowledgment and validation) can perpetuate chronic pain. In Australia, for example, many academics feel that the coining of RSI as a diagnostic term, as well as the government's early move to provide compensation for the illness as a work-related handicap, triggered the epidemic. When the diagnosis fell out of favour with physicians and disability coverage became more difficult to get, the number of symptoms associated with the disorder decreased. It also appeared that initial exposure regarding the potential causes of arm pain, as well as active attempts in some areas to improve arm pain reporting or implement ergonomic adjustments, merely exacerbated the epidemic. More recently, in the United States, there has been a discussion about the roots of a comparable workplace epidemic known as repetitive-stress injury, repetitive-motion disorder, and—in the present nomenclature—cumulative-trauma disorder. Once again, the most significant risk factors appear to be social rather than physical.

Back and arm discomfort are not alone in having nonphysical reasons. According to research, social factors play a significant influence in many chronic-pain syndromes, including chronic pelvic pain, temporomandibular joint disease, and chronic tension headache. Again, none of this suggests that people are faking it. According to Melzack's view, pain that does not result from physical harm is just as genuine as pain that does—in the brain, the two are identical. As a result, taking a compassionate approach to chronic pain entails looking into its social as well as physical dimensions. The solution to chronic pain may lay in what happens around us rather than what happens inside us. Of all the implications of the new pain theory, this one appears to be the strangest and most far-reaching: it has turned pain political.

Chapter 8: A Queasy Feeling

Fitzpatrick was twenty-nine years old, tall, with long, thick black hair set against pale Irish skin and a dimpled, almost juvenile face that made it difficult for others to take her seriously, despite her Wharton MBA. She lived in Manhattan with her husband, an investment banker, and commuted to Manhasset, Long Island, where she worked as a management consultant for North Shore Health System. It was a brisk March morning, and she wanted to locate a place to stop quickly.

Her stomach was rolling when she stepped off the F.D.R. onto the slope leading to the Triborough Bridge. She was in what experts refer to as the "prodromal phase of emesis." Salivation increases, often in torrential fashion. The pupils dilated. The heart starts to race. The blood vessels in the skin constrict, causing pallor—NASA scientists have even utilised skin sensors to detect space sickness in astronauts, who are frequently hesitant to admit to feeling ill. People break into a chilly sweat. Fatigue and drowsiness typically appear within minutes. Attention, reflexes, and concentration fade.

While all of this is happening, the stomach experiences aberrant electrical activity, preventing it from emptying and causing it to relax. The oesophagus contracts, drawing the top portion of the stomach from the belly, up the diaphragm, and into the chest, creating a funnel from stomach to oesophagus. In a single movement known as the "retrograde giant contraction," the upper small intestine evacuates its contents backward into the stomach, preparing for vomiting. Smaller rhythmic contractions in the lower small intestine drive materials toward the colon.

As Fitzpatrick exited the ramp, the lanes spread out like a fan, and all the drivers around her jockeyed for place. She looked for a spot to pull over on the right side of the road, but there wasn't one. She began to cut across the lanes to the left, aiming for a no-man's land between traffic entering the toll booths and traffic exiting in the opposite direction. She started retching and pulled out an empty plastic grocery bag. Then she vomited. Some puke got on her outfit and jacket. Some got into the bag she was holding with one hand. She kept her eyes open and the car steady, however, and managed to get out of the jam. Then she came to a standstill, bent forward against her shoulder belt, and retrieved whatever she had left.

Vomiting normally makes people feel better, at least for a short time, but Fitzpatrick felt no better. She sat there with the cars flying by, hoping the sick feeling would leave, but it didn't. Still uneasy, she drove over the bridge, turned around, returned home, and climbed into bed. Over the next few days, she began to lose her appetite, and strong odours became unbearable. That Easter weekend, she and her husband, Bob, drove to Alexandria, Virginia, to visit her relatives. She was hardly able to bear the travel and had to spend it lying flat in the back seat. It would take months before she could return to New York.

At her parents' house, her symptoms immediately worsened. She couldn't keep any food or liquids down that weekend. She became completely dehydrated. She spent a few hours in the hospital on the Monday following Easter, receiving intravenous fluids. She saw her mother's obstetrician, who reassured her that nausea and vomiting were normal during pregnancy and gave her some common, practical advice: avoid strong odours and cold liquids, and eat small amounts of food whenever possible, such as dry crackers and other carbohydrates. Fitzpatrick's symptoms were normal, thus the doctor did not want to prescribe anything. She pointed out that pregnancy sickness normally goes away by the fourteenth or sixteenth week of pregnancy.

What is nausea, this strange and terrifying creature? Despite receiving little attention in medical school, nausea is the most common ailment for which individuals contact physicians, second only to pain. It's a common side effect of medications. Vomiting after anaesthesia is so common in surgery patients that a "emesis basin" is maintained by each bed in the recovery area. The majority of chemotherapy patients experience nausea, which they regularly regard as the worst aspect of the treatment. Morning sickness, sometimes known as "pregnancy sickness," affects 60 to 85 percent of pregnant women, and it causes one-third of those who work to miss work. In around five out of every thousand pregnant women, the illness is severe enough to cause significant weight loss—a condition known as "hyperemesis of pregnancy." And, of course, almost everyone has motion sickness at some point in their lives. Seasickness has been a key military concern since ancient Greece. (The word nausea is derived from the Greek word for ship.) Cybersickness continues to impede the development of virtual reality technologies. And space sickness is a common, but rarely discussed, issue for astronauts.

The most noticeable aspect of nausea is how deeply unpleasant it is (Cicero declared he "would rather be killed than again suffer the tortures of seasickness"), and not simply in the moment. Long after the pain of labour has faded from memory, moms will clearly recall their nausea; it is even one of the reasons why some women do not wish to have further children. Nausea is remarkable in this regard. Break a leg on a ski hill, and—as painful as it is—you will ski again. In contrast, after one bad experience with a bottle of gin or an oyster, individuals avoid the perpetrator for years. In Anthony Burgess's A Clockwork Orange, the government programmed Alex to avoid cruelty by associating his violent tendencies with nausea rather than pain. At one point, some German towns made similar initiatives. According to an 1843 manuscript, disobedient teenagers were placed inside a box outside town hall, after which a police officer whirled the box around at high speed until the youngsters had offered the gathered crowd with a "disgusting spectacle."

Nausea and vomiting appear to have a biological purpose despite their unpleasantness. The benefit of vomiting after eating dangerous or poisoned food is obvious: the toxin is eliminated. And the horrible nausea makes you never want to eat anything like that again. This explains why medications, chemotherapy, and general anaesthetics frequently cause nausea and vomiting: they are poisons—albeit regulated ones—that the body is programmed to reject.

Why other items trigger nausea and vomiting is harder to explain, but scientists are starting to find some logic in nature's design. Pregnancy illness, for example, would appear to be evolutionary detrimental, given that a growing embryo needs nutrients. In a well-known 1992 publication, evolutionary biologist Margie Profet established a persuasive case that pregnant illness is actually protective. She stated that natural foods that are acceptable for adults are often hazardous for embryos. All plants produce poisons, and in order to consume them, mammals have evolved complex detoxifying systems. However, these systems can not completely eliminate hazardous substances, and embryos can be susceptible to even trace levels. (Toxins in potatoes, for example, have been discovered to cause brain deformities in animal foetuses, even at levels that are benign to their mothers; fact, Ireland's high rate of neural abnormalities, such as spina bifida, may be attributed to its excessive potato diet.)

The Prophet hypothesised that pregnancy illness evolved to protect an embryo from natural poisons. She stated that ladies suffering from pregnancy sickness prefer bland foods that do not decay quickly (such as breads and cereals) and are especially wary of items high in natural toxins, such as bitter or spicy foods and animal products that are not exceptionally fresh. The theory also explains why nausea occurs primarily in the first trimester. That is when the embryo develops organs and is most sensitive to toxins; nevertheless, it is small, and its calorie requirements are easily met by the mother's fat stores. Women with moderate to severe morning sickness have a decreased risk of miscarriage than women with mild nausea or none at all.

Regardless of how adaptive nausea and vomiting are, in cases of hyperemesis such as Amy Fitzpatrick's, these reflexes appear to spin out of control. Indeed, until World War II and the invention of current fluid replacement procedures, hyperemesis was almost always fatal unless the pregnancy was aborted. Even today, although mortality is rare, excessive vomiting can cause catastrophic harm, including esophageal rupture, lung collapse, and spleen tearing. Nobody would argue that Fitzpatrick's situation was in the least favourable. Something needed to be done to aid her.

Fitzpatrick's doctor prescribed medicines when she lost twelve pounds in order to control her nausea and vomiting and allow her to eat and drink again. The doctor first tried Reglan, a medication commonly used to relieve nausea caused by general anaesthesia. Fitzpatrick wore a gadget that injected the medicine into her leg around the clock. It didn't appear to help, though; instead, it caused terrifying neurological side effects like tremors, lockjaw, body rigidity, and difficulties breathing. The doctor tried a second medicine, Compazine, which did not help much, and then another, Phenergan suppositories, which made her drowsy but did not stop the vomiting.

All of these medicines function by inhibiting dopamine receptors in the brain. However, there is a newer class of antiemetics on the market today: serotonin-receptor blockers, which have been heralded as a breakthrough in nausea and vomiting treatment. They aren't cheap—Zofran, the best-selling medication, costing $125 a day or more—but studies show that they significantly reduce vomiting in chemotherapy patients and some surgery patients. No concerns with birth abnormalities have been identified. Fitzpatrick was given Zofran intravenously for several weeks, but to no result.

Meanwhile, a small group of family and friends meticulously gathered information on both traditional and alternative therapy alternatives. Fitzpatrick experimented with herbal therapy, Chinese massage, and lemon water at different times. She tried ginger after learning about a study that suggested it would be beneficial for her illness. She tried Sea-Bands, which are acupressure bracelets that provide consistent pressure to the "Neiguan point" on the inside of each forearm, three finger-widths down from the wrist crease and between the tendons. (Acupressure has been advertised as a treatment for nausea caused by pregnancy, chemotherapy, and motion, but studies have found no consistent impact.) None of it helped Fitzpatrick's nausea, though she did love the massages. Even more concerning, her symptoms were not improving with time, as her doctors had predicted. By the fourth month of her pregnancy, she was as nauseous as she had ever been—a highly unusual occurrence. She appeared frighteningly unwell. Her weight went down sixteen pounds. Her doctor admitted her to George Washington University Hospital and scheduled an appointment with the high-risk obstetrics unit. She was put on intravenous feeding and finally began to gain weight. During the next six months, however, she spent more time in the hospital than outside.

To her doctors, she was now a phantom, ever-present reminder of failure—the type of patient whose mere existence is a disgrace to them and their skill. Doctors have numerous approaches to dealing with these people, and she must have encountered them all. Some doctors assured her that she would recover in a week or two. One doctor inquired if she wanted to return to New York, and she had the unmistakable sensation that he only wanted to get rid of her. Another person seemed to think she wasn't trying hard enough to eat, as if the sickness was under her control. Their displeasure was evident. Later, they suggested she consult a psychiatrist. This wasn't an unreasonable proposal. Anxiety and worry may cause nausea, so she was eager to try anything that would help. However, Fitzpatrick claims that the psychiatrist who visited her continued to focus on whether she was furious with the babies and unable to accept her duties as wife and mother. A surprising percentage of clinicians continue to believe the erroneous Freudian hypothesis that hyperemesis is caused by an unconscious rejection of pregnancy.

There is no universal antiemetic. Scopolamine-containing skin patches prevent motion sickness and postoperative vomiting, although they appear to be ineffective for pregnant women and chemotherapy patients. The dopamine-receptor antagonist Phenergan is effective for many pregnant women and motion sickness sufferers, but not for chemotherapy patients. Even cutting-edge drugs like Zofran, which is commonly regarded as a type of penicillin for nausea, are frequently ineffective. While Zofran is particularly effective against chemotherapy and anaesthesia-induced vomiting, research demonstrates that it does not help with motion sickness or pregnant hyperemesis. (Smoking marijuana appears to be useful for chemotherapy patients, albeit faintly, but it is just as hazardous to the foetus during pregnancy as tobacco.)

This makes sense when you consider that nausea can be provoked by a variety of triggers, including an unusual motion, a foul scent, a poisonous medicine, and pregnancy hormone swings. According to scientists, the brain has a vomiting program (or "module") that receives and responds to a variety of inputs, including chemoreceptors in the nose, gut, and brain; receptors that detect stomach overfilling or uvula tickling; motion sensors in the inner ear; and higher brain centres that govern memory, mood, and cognition. Each of our existing medications appears to interfere with some pathways more than others. As a result, the consequences differ depending on the condition.

Researchers examining chemotherapy patients, who serve as a captive population for scientists studying how nausea and vomiting occur, uncovered something even more shocking. These patients suffer three distinct types of nausea and vomiting. An "acute" kind develops within minutes to hours of getting a deadly chemotherapy treatment and then progressively resolves—exactly the response we would expect from a toxin. However, in many cases, the nausea and vomiting return after a day or two, a phenomenon known as "delayed emesis." Approximately a quarter of chemotherapy patients experience "anticipatory nausea and vomiting," which occurs before the medicines are injected. Morrow has identified some distinguishing features of various types of nausea. The stronger the initial acute nausea, the worse the anticipatory nausea grows. And the more cycles of chemotherapy that patients receive, the more general the cues for anticipatory nausea become: vomiting may occur first when a patient sees the nurse who administers the drugs, then when he sees any nurse or smells the clinic, and finally when he drives into the clinic parking lot for his chemotherapy appointment. One of Morrow's patients vomited anytime she saw the hospital's highway exit sign.

Ultimately, our medicinal armament against nausea and vomiting remains rather basic. Given how widespread these issues are and how much people are ready to pay to have them resolved, pharmaceutical companies are investing millions of dollars in research to develop more effective medications. Merck, for example, has produced a potential candidate, known as MK-869. This is one of a new family of drugs known as "substance P antagonists." These medications drew a lot of interest when Merck stated that they appeared to be clinically effective against depression. Less well known, however, were studies published in the New England Journal of Medicine suggesting MK-869 was exceptionally effective against nausea and vomiting in chemotherapy patients.

The results were unexpected for two reasons. First, the medication significantly reduced acute and delayed vomiting. Second, MK-869 not only prevented vomiting but also reduced nausea. The medication reduced the proportion of patients reporting anything more than mild nausea in the five days following chemotherapy from 75% to 51%.

All of our therapies have limitations, and no matter how promising these new drugs appear, they will fail many people. Not even MK-869 could alleviate nausea in half of chemotherapy patients. (Additionally, its safety and effectiveness in pregnant women are likely to be unclear for some time. Because of both medical and legal risks, drug companies generally avoid testing medications on pregnant women. So there is no morphine for nausea in the future. Uncontrolled nausea is a persistent problem. Still, a brand-new clinical specialty known as "palliative medicine" is pursuing a bold goal: the scientific study of suffering. And what's interesting is that they're discovering solutions where others haven't.

Palliative care specialists are experts in caring for dying patients, with a focus on increasing their quality of life rather than prolonging it. One would say we don't need a specialty for this, but there is evidence that these specialists are indeed better at it. Dying patients frequently experience pain. Many people have nausea. Some people have such low lung function that, despite taking in enough oxygen to survive, they experience persistent, terrible breathlessness—a feeling like they are drowning and can't get enough air. These are people with incurable diseases, yet palliative care doctors have been remarkably effective in helping them. The issue is that they consider suffering to be a problem in and of itself. In medicine, we're accustomed to viewing such symptoms as clues in a puzzle about where the disease is and what we can do about it. And, in most cases, removing the infected appendix, setting the broken bone, or treating the pneumonia is the most effective strategy to alleviate suffering. (I wouldn't be a surgeon if I believed otherwise.) However, this is not always the case, and nausea is a prime example. Most of the time, nausea is not an indication of disease, but rather a normal reaction to something like travel or pregnancy—or even a useful treatment like chemotherapy, antibiotics, or general anaesthesia. We say the patient is "fine," but the agony is just as severe.

Perhaps the most remarkable observation made by palliative care doctors is that there is a separation between symptom and pain. According to physician Eric J. Cassell in his book The Nature of Suffering and the Goals of Medicine, for some patients, simply receiving a measure of understanding—knowing what the source of the misery is, seeing its meaning in a different way, or simply accepting that we cannot always tame nature—can be sufficient to control their suffering. Even if your meds have failed, a doctor can still help.

Amy Fitzpatrick claimed that the doctors she loved best were the ones that admitted they didn't know what was causing her sickness or how to treat it. They would claim they had never seen anything like her condition, and she could sense they sympathised with her. She acknowledged having conflicting thoughts regarding such admissions. They made her worry if she was seeing the appropriate doctors, or if they were missing something. However, no matter what remedies she and the doctors attempted, the nausea persisted. It truly seemed beyond anyone's comprehension.

The first few months were a hard, frightening struggle. However, she gradually sensed a transformation, a toughening of her soul, and she occasionally had the impression that things weren't so horrible after all. She prayed every day and believed that the two children growing inside her were a gift from God, and over time, she grew to see her struggles as simply the cost of such incredible joy. She gave up searching for silver bullets. She requested that no further experimental therapies be performed beyond the twenty-sixth week of pregnancy. The nausea and vomiting persisted, but she refused to be overcome by them.

There was finally some relief. By the third week, she had discovered that she could eat an unusual combination of four things in silver-size portions: steak, asparagus, tuna, and mint ice cream. She also managed to keep a protein drink down. The nausea persisted, although it had subsided only little. Fitzpatrick went into active labour at the thirty-third week, seven weeks before schedule. Her husband arrived at the delivery location on time via shuttle from LaGuardia. The physicians had warned her that the twins would be little, weighing approximately three pounds, but Linda was delivered on September 12 at 10:52 p.m., weighing four pounds and twelve ounces. Jack was born at five pounds, both in perfect condition.

Chapter 9: Crimson Tide

Christine Drury took over as the overnight anchorwoman for Channel 13 News, Indianapolis' local NBC station, in January 1997. This is how to get started in television news and chat shows. (David Letterman began his career doing weekend weather for the same station.) Drury worked the 9 p.m. to 5 a.m. shift, crafting articles and reading bulletins after midnight. If she was lucky and there was breaking news in the middle of the night, she could obtain more airtime by reporting the story live, either from the newsroom or on the ground. If she was exceptionally lucky—like when a Conrail train crashed in Greencastle—she'd be able to stay for the morning show. During her broadcasts, however, she discovered that she could not stop blushing. The slightest insignificant event was sufficient to set things off. She'd be on set, reading the news, and suddenly stumble over a word or realise she was speaking too quickly. She became red very instantly. A sensation of electric heat would begin in her breast and spread upward to her neck, ears, and scalp. In physiological terms, it was just a redirection of blood flow. The face and neck have an unusually large number of veins at the surface, which can carry more blood than veins of comparable size elsewhere. When stimulated by particular neurological signals, they expand while other peripheral veins contract, causing the hands to turn white and clammy as the face flushes. More worrisome for Drury than the physical reaction was the distress that came with it: her thoughts would go blank, and she'd hear herself stammering. She would have an overpowering need to cover her face with her hands, turn away from the camera, and hide.

Drury had been a blusher since she could remember, and her pale Irish skin made her flushes stand out. She was the type of child who almost always blushed with shame when called on in class or while looking for a seat in the lunchroom. As an adult, she could be embarrassed by a grocery store cashier holding up the line to get a price on her cornflakes, or by being honked at while driving. It may appear weird that such a person would pose in front of a camera. But Drury had always overcome her desire to be embarrassed. In high school, she was a cheerleader, a tennis player, and a prom queen. She had participated in intramural tennis, rowing crew with friends, and graduated Phi Beta Kappa while at Purdue. She had previously worked as a server and assistant manager at a Wal-Mart, leading the staff in the Wal-Mart cheer every morning. Her outgoing personality and social elegance had always ensured her a vast group of acquaintances.

Drury gave up caffeine. She attempted breath-control techniques. She purchased self-help books for television actors and assumed the camera was her puppy, a friend, or her mother. She tried holding her head a certain manner, very still, while on camera. Nothing worked.

Being an overnight anchor is not a particularly appealing job due to the long hours and limited exposure. People often work for around a year, perfecting their skills before moving on to a better position. But Drury wasn't going anywhere. "She was definitely not ready to be on during daylight hours," the producer explained. In October 1998, over two years into her career, she wrote in her journal, "My sensations of slipping persist. I cried all day. I'm on my way to work and feel like I'll never have enough Kleenex. I don't see why God would give me a job I can't do. I need to figure out how to do this. I will try everything before giving up."

But if we're worried about shame, why do we blush when we get compliments? Or when they sing "Happy Birthday" to us? Or when they simply glance at us? Michael Lewis, a professor of psychiatry at the University of Medicine and Dentistry of New Jersey, frequently displays the effect in class. He says that he will randomly point at a pupil, that the pointing is meaningless and does not reflect any judgement on the person. He then closes his eyes and points. Everyone checks to see who it is. Invariably, such a person is overtaken with embarrassment. In an unusual experiment conducted a few years ago, two social psychologists, Janice Templeton and Mark Leary, wired individuals with facial-temperature sensors and placed them on one side of a one-way mirror. The mirror was then removed, revealing a large audience staring at them from the opposite side. Half of the audience members wore dark glasses, half did not. Surprisingly, individuals reddened only when they noticed the audience's eyes.

The most worrisome aspect of blushing is that it has secondary effects of its own. It is embarrassing and can result in acute self-consciousness, bewilderment, and lack of attention. (Darwin, unable to explain why this occurred, hypothesised that increased blood supply to the face drained blood from the brain.)

In the fall of 1998, Drury went to see an internist. "You'll grow out of it," he told her. When she pressed, however, he agreed to let her try medication. It couldn't have been obvious what to prescribe. Medical textbooks say nothing about pathological blushing. Some doctors prescribe anxiolytics, like Valium, on the assumption that the real problem is anxiety. Some prescribe beta-blockers, which blunt the body's stress response. Some prescribe Prozac or other antidepressants. The one therapy that has been shown to have modest success is not a drug but a behavioural technique known as paradoxical intention—having patients actively try to blush instead of trying not to. Drury used beta-blockers first, then antidepressants, and finally psychotherapy. There was no improvement.

By December 1998, her blushing had become unbearable, her on-air performance humiliating, and her career nearly irreparable. She wrote in her diary that she was prepared to resign. Then one day, she searched the Internet for information on facial blushing and came across a facility in Sweden where doctors were doing a surgical operation to stop it. The procedure entailed severing particular nerves in the chest where they exit the spinal cord and travel up to the head.

Drury decided to spend some time learning more about the surgery. She read the few papers available in medical journals. She chatted with the surgeons and previous patients. After a few weeks, she became even more convinced. She told her parents she was going to Sweden, and when it became evident she would not be dissuaded, her father agreed to accompany her. The procedure is known as endoscopic thoracic sympathectomy, or ETS. It entails removing fibres of a person's sympathetic nervous system, which is a subset of the involuntary, or "autonomic," neural system that regulates respiration, heart rate, digestion, perspiration, and, among many other basic activities, blushing. The sympathetic trunks, which run down either side of the spine like two smooth white strings, are located in the back of your chest. They serve as access roads for sympathetic nerves before they exit to various organs. At the turn of the twentieth century, surgeons attempted to remove branches of these trunks—a thoracic sympathectomy—for a variety of ailments, including epilepsy, glaucoma, and certain types of blindness. Most of the tests caused more harm than good. However, surgeons discovered two exceptional cases in which a sympathectomy helped: it relieved intractable chest discomfort in patients with advanced, inoperable cardiac disease, and it eliminated hand and facial sweating in patients with hyperhidrosis (uncontrollable sweating).

The operation is currently performed all around the world, however the Göteborg surgeons are among the few who have published their findings: 94 percent of their patients reported a significant reduction in blushing, with most cases totally eradicated. In polls conducted eight months after the surgery, 2 percent regretted the decision due to side effects, while 15% were dissatisfied. The adverse effects are not life-threatening, but they are not minor. Homer's syndrome, which occurs in 1% of patients, is the most devastating injury, characterised by a constricted pupil, drooping eyelid, and sunken eyeball caused by unintended damage to the sympathetic nerves that supply the eye. Less seriously, patients no longer sweat from the nipples up, and the majority perceive a significant increase in lower-body perspiration as a result. (A longer-term research that examined hand-sweating patients a decade after getting ETS found that the number of patients who were satisfied with the outcome dropped to only 67 percent, owing primarily to compensatory sweating.) Approximately one-third of patients experience gustatory sweating, which is perspiration induced by specific tastes or scents. Furthermore, because sympathetic branches to the heart are eliminated, patients suffer a 10% drop in heart rate; some report poor physical performance. For all of these reasons, doctors believe that the operation should only be used as a last resort, after all other options have failed. By the time people call Göteborg, they are frequently desperate.

On January 14, 1999, Christine Drury and her father came to Göteborg. The city is a four-hundred-year-old seaport on Sweden's southwest coast, and she recalls the weather as cold, snowy, and lovely. The Carlanderska Medical Center was old and modest, with ivy-covered walls and large arched wooden double doors. Inside, it was dim and silent, reminding Drury of a dungeon. Only now did she grow concerned, wondering what she was doing here, nine thousand miles from home, at a hospital she knew little about. Nonetheless, she signed in, and a nurse drew her blood for normal lab testing, verified her medical papers, and received her payment, which totaled $6,000. Drury placed it on his credit card.

An orderly arrived at nine thirty that morning to take her to the operating room. While Drury was unconscious, Drott, dressed in scrubs and a sterile gown, swabbed her chest and axillae (underarms) with antiseptic and set down sterile drapes to expose only her axillae. He felt a gap between the ribs in her left axilla and made a seven-millimetre puncture with the tip of his scalpel before pushing a large-bore needle through it and into her chest. Two litres of carbon dioxide were injected through the needle, pushing her left lung down and out of the way. Drott then inserted a resectoscope, which is a long metal tube with an eyepiece, fibre-optic light, and a cauterising tip. It is actually a urological equipment that may pass through the urethra. Looking through the lens, he searched for her left sympathetic trunk, being careful not to injure her heart's main blood veins, and discovered the glabrous, cordlike tissue resting along the tops of her ribs, where they meet the spine. He cauterised the trunk at two locations, over the second and third ribs, destroying all facial branches except those leading to the eye. After ensuring that there was no bleeding, he removed the instrument and inserted a catheter to suck out the carbon dioxide and allow her lung to re-expand before suturing the quarter-inch incision. Moving to the opposite side of the table, he repeated the process on her right chest. Everything went smoothly. The procedure took only twenty minutes.

Almost two years after Drury's procedure, I saw her for lunch at an Indianapolis sports bar. I was wondering what her face would look like without the nerves that control its colour—would she seem ashen, blotchy, or strange in some way? In truth, her face is clear and a little reddish, as she previously stated. She hasn't blushed since the procedure. She has occasionally, almost randomly, encountered a phantom blush, which is the unmistakable impression that she is blushing when she is not. I inquired if her face reddened while she ran, and she responded no, but it would if she stood on her head. The other bodily changes appeared insignificant to her. The most visible difference, she stated, was that neither her face nor her arms sweated anymore, while her stomach, back, and legs sweated significantly more than before, but not enough to annoy her. The scars, which were minor to begin with, have completely faded. Drury claims she felt altered from the first morning following the operation. A beautiful nurse arrived to check her blood pressure. Normally, she would have blushed the moment he approached. But nothing of the sort occurred. She felt as if a mask had been removed.

That day, after being discharged, she put herself to the test by asking random strangers on the street for directions, which always made her blush. Now, her father has confirmed, she did not. Furthermore, the encounters felt natural and ordinary, with no trace of her previous self-consciousness. She recalls being at the airport with her father, waiting in a long check-in queue, and being unable to locate her passport. Back home, everything looked new. Attention no longer felt complex or terrifying. Her customary internal monologue when speaking with others ("Please don't blush, please don't blush, oh God, I'm going to blush") vanished, and she discovered that she could listen to others more effectively. She could also look at them for extended periods of time without feeling compelled to turn away. (She had to train herself to stop staring.)

Later, I saw some records of her broadcasts from the first several weeks after the surgery. I saw her report on a drunk driver killing a local priest, as well as a sixteen-year-old shooting a 19-year-old. She was as natural as she had ever been. One specific broadcast touched me. It wasn't her usual evening briefing, but a public service announcement dubbed "Read, Indiana, Read!" On a February morning, she was shown reading a story to a group of obstreperous eight-year-olds while messages encouraging parents to read to their children scrolled by. Despite the commotion of children walking by, throwing stuff, and putting their faces up to the camera, she remained poised throughout.

Drury had kept the operation a secret, but her coworkers noticed a difference right away. I spoke with a producer at her station, who stated, "She just told me she was going on a trip with her father, but when she returned and I saw her on TV again, I said, 'Christine! That was unbelievable!'" She appeared incredibly at ease in front of the camera. You could sense the confidence coming through the television, which was really different from previously." Within months, Drury secured a position as a prime-time on-air reporter at another station.

A few fibre snips to her face and she was transformed. It's a weird concept because we think of our essential self as separate from such physical details. Who hasn't looked at a snapshot of themselves or heard their voice on audio and thought, "That isn't me!" To give an extreme example, burn patients who see themselves in a mirror for the first time often feel alienated by their looks. But they don't just "get used" to it; their new skin transforms them. It affects how individuals interact with others, what they anticipate from others, and how they perceive themselves in the eyes of others. A burn-ward nurse once told me that the secure might become afraid and spiteful, while the weak can become jut-jawed "survivors." Similarly, Drury had perceived her trip-wire blushing as something wholly external, similar to a burn—"the red mask," as she referred to it. However, it penetrated so deeply within her that she believed it kept her from becoming the person she was destined to be. Once the disguise was removed, she appeared new, bold, and "completely different from before." But what about the individual who has spent her entire life feeling ashamed and self-conscious at the slightest scrutiny? That individual, Drury eventually realised, was still present.

On television, self-consciousness began to distract her once more. She began her new position in June 1999, although she was not slated to appear on TV for another two months. During the sabbatical, she became unsure about returning to television. One day that summer, she went out with a crew to cover storm damage in a nearby town where trees had been uprooted. They allowed her to practise her stand-up routine in front of the camera. She was certain she looked fine, but that was not how she felt. "I felt like I didn't belong there, didn't deserve to be there," she tells me. Several days later, she resigned.

More than a year has gone since then, and Drury has had to use that time to get her life back on track. Unemployed and ashamed, she withdrew, saw no one, and spent her days watching TV from her couch, sinking deeper into misery. Her situation changed gradually. Against her better judgement, she began telling friends and later former coworkers what had transpired. To her astonishment and relief, almost everyone was encouraging. In September 1999, she founded the Red Mask Foundation to raise awareness of chronic blushing and create a support network for those affected. Revealing her secret seemed to help her move on.

That winter, she landed a new job in radio, which made perfect sense. She became the assistant bureau chief for Metro Networks radio in Indianapolis. Every weekday morning, she could be heard anchoring the news on two radio stations, followed by the afternoon traffic report for these and several additional stations. Last spring, after regaining her confidence, she began contacting television stations. The local Fox station agreed to let her serve as a substitute announcer. In early July, she was called in at the last minute to handle traffic for the three-hour morning show. I got to view the show on videotape. It was one of those breakfast news shows with two cheerful co-anchors—a man and a woman—sitting in plush chairs, holding massive coffee mugs. Every half hour or so, they'd ask Drury for a two-minute traffic report. She'd stand in front of a series of projected city maps, scrolling among them and outlining the numerous vehicle accidents and construction obstacles to watch for. The co-anchors would occasionally engage in some hey-you-aren't-our-usual-traffic-gal banter, which she handled well, laughing and joking. It was exciting, she admits, but not easy. She couldn't help but feel self-conscious about returning after such a long hiatus. But the emotions did not overpower her. She claims she's starting to feel more at ease with herself.

Chapter 10: The Man Who Couldn't Stop Eating

A Roux-en-Y gastric bypass surgery is a radical technique and the most dramatic way to lose weight. It is also the strangest surgical procedure in which I have ever participated. It does not cure sickness, fix defects, or heal injuries. It is a surgery designed to manage a person's will—to manipulate a person's internal organs so that he does not overeat again. And it is rapidly gaining popularity. In 1999, over 45,000 obese people underwent gastric bypass surgery in the United States, with the figure expected to double by 2003. Vincent Caselli was going to join them.

On September 13, 1999, at 7:30 a.m., an anesthesiologist and two orderlies led Caselli (whose name has been changed) to the operating room, where I and his attending surgeon awaited him. Caselli was fifty-four years old, a heavy-machine operator and road construction contractor (he and his workers had paved a rotary in my area), the son of Italian immigrants, a husband of thirty-five years, and a father to three daughters, all of whom were now adults with their own families. He also weighed 428 pounds despite being only 5'7" tall, and he was miserable. He was housebound, and his health was declining, so he no longer lived a regular existence.

He was the mountain on the table. I'm six feet two, but even with the table as low as it goes, I had to stand on a step stool to operate; Dr. Randall used two stools piled together. He nodded, and I cut into the centre of our patient's belly, through skin and dense inches of shimmering yellow fat. Inside his belly, his liver was stained with fat, and his intestines were wrapped in a thick apron, but his stomach appeared normal—a smooth, greyish-pink sack the size of two hands. We used metal retractors to keep the wound open and the liver and intestinal loops out of the way. Working elbow deep, we stapled his stomach to the size of an ounce. Before the operation, it could carry a quart of food and drink; today it can only hold a shot glass. We next connected the opening of this little pouch to a section of his colon two feet beyond his duodenum—past the first segment of the small bowel, where bile and pancreatic juices break down food. This was the bypass aspect of the operation, which meant that any food the stomach could hold would be less easily digested.

We spent little more than two hours performing the operation. Caselli remained steady throughout, but his recuperation proved challenging. Patients are often discharged three days after surgery; Caselli had no idea where he was for two days. For twenty-four hours, his kidneys stopped working, and fluid accumulated in his lungs. He grew crazy, seeing objects on the walls, removing his oxygen mask, chest leads for the monitors, and even ripping out the IV in his arm. We were frightened, and his wife and girls were afraid, but he eventually pulled through.

By the third day after surgery, he was able to drink up to one ounce of clear liquids each four hours. During my afternoon rounds, I asked him how the sips went down. "OK," he said. We started giving him four-ounce servings of Carnation Instant Breakfast for protein and fewer calories. He could barely finish half, and it took him an hour. It filled him full, causing a sharp, uncomfortable discomfort. This was to be expected, Dr. Randall informed him. It will take a few days before he is ready for solid food. But he was doing fine. He no longer needed intravenous fluids. The agony from his injuries was under control. And, after a brief stint in a rehabilitation facility, we returned him home.

Vincent Caselli and his wife reside in a modest saltbox home not far from Boston. To get there, I drove along Route 1, passing four Dunkin' Donuts, four pizzerias, three steak places, two McDonald's, two Ground Rounds, a Taco Bell, a Friendly's, and an International House of Pancakes. (A regular roadside view, but on that particular day it appeared to be a sombre tour of our self-destructive tendencies.) I pressed the doorbell, and a long minute passed. I heard a sluggish footfall approaching the door, and Caselli, clearly exhausted, opened it. But when he spotted me, he grinned broadly and squeezed my hand gently. He guided me to a breakfast table in his flowered-wallpaper kitchen, resting his hand on the table, wall, and door jamb for stability.

We talked about his return home from the hospital. His first solid meal experience was a tablespoon of scrambled eggs. Just that amount made him so full that it hurt, he added, "like something was ripping," and he spewed it up again. He was concerned that nothing concrete would ever come down. He eventually discovered that he could handle small amounts of soft meals, such as mashed potatoes, macaroni, and even chicken if finely chopped and moist. Breads and dry meats, he discovered, became "stuck," requiring him to insert a finger down his throat and force himself to vomit.

Caselli was unhappy that things had come to this, but he had accepted the necessity of the situation. "The last year or two, I've been in hell," he remarked. The conflict had started in his late twenties. "I always had some weight on me," he admitted. He weighed 200 pounds when he married Teresa (as I'll call her), and 300 pounds a decade later. He'd diet and drop 75 pounds, then regain 100. By 1985, he weighed 400 pounds. On one diet, he lost a hundred and ninety pounds. Then he shot up again. "I must have gained and lost a thousand pounds," I heard him say. He got excessive blood pressure, elevated cholesterol, and diabetes. His legs and back aches all the time. He had limited movement. He used to acquire season tickets to Boston Bruins games and visit the Seekonk racetrack every summer to watch motor racing. Years ago, he raced himself. Now he could barely walk to his pickup truck. He hadn't been on an aeroplane since 1983, and he hadn't been to the second story of his own house in two years due to his inability to handle the stairs. "Teresa bought a computer a year ago for her office upstairs, and I've never seen it," he said. He had to relocate from their bedroom upstairs to a little room off the kitchen. He couldn't lie down and has been sleeping in a recliner ever since. Despite this, he could only sleep in snatches due to sleep apnea, a frequent syndrome among obese people that is considered to be caused by extra fat in the tongue and soft tissues of the upper airway. Every thirty minutes, his respiration would cease, and he'd awaken asphyxiated. He was always fatigued.

There were other issues, the kind that few people talk about. Good hygiene, he claimed, was practically impossible. He could no longer stand to urinate, and after emptying his bowels, he frequently had to shower to get clean. Skin creases would become chafed and red, with occasional boils and infections. "Has it been a strain on your marriage?" I requested an answer. "Sure," he replied. "Sex life is nonexistent. I have high hopes for it. For him, the worst thing was his declining ability to earn a living.

Vincent Caselli's father moved to Boston from Italy in 1914 to work in construction. He quickly obtained five steam shovels and started his own business. Vince and his brother took over the firm in the 1960s, and Vince ventured out on his own in 1979. He was an expert at operating heavy equipment—his specialty was driving a Gradall, a thirty-ton, three-hundred-thousand-dollar hydraulic excavator—and he hired a team of men year-round to create roads and walkways. He eventually bought his own Gradall, a ten-wheel Mack dump truck, a backhoe, and a collection of pickup trucks. But, during the last three years, he had grown too large to run the Gradall or keep up with the daily upkeep of the equipment. He had to handle the firm from his home and pay people to do the heavy lifting; he enlisted a nephew to assist with the men and contracts. Expenses grew, and because he could no longer make the rounds of city halls on his own, obtaining contracts became increasingly difficult. They would have gone bankrupt if Teresa's employment, as business manager for an assisted-living home in Boston, had not saved them.

As far as I could tell, Caselli ate for the same reasons that everyone else does: food tasted good, it was seven o'clock and time for supper, and a wonderful meal had been prepared on the table. And he stopped eating for the same reason everyone does: he was full and it was no longer enjoyable. The biggest difference seems to be that he needed an unusual amount of food to be satisfied. (He could finish a huge pizza without blinking.) To lose weight, he had to do the same arduous work that every dieter does: quit eating before he was full, while the food still tasted delicious, and exercise. These were things he could perform for a short time, and possibly longer with some reminders and coaching, but they were not something he could do for very long. "I am not strong," he said.

In early 1998, Caselli's internist advised him severely, "If you can't lose this weight, we'll have to do something drastic." And by this, she meant surgery. She detailed the gastric bypass procedure to him and offered him Dr. Randall's phone number. Caselli refused to consider it. The process itself was bad enough. He couldn't put his business on hold for that. A year later, in the spring of 1999, he suffered serious infections in both legs: as his weight climbed and varicosities emerged, the skin thinned and deteriorated, resulting in open, purulent ulcers. Despite fevers and excruciating discomfort, he finally consented to attend his doctor after his wife persisted in convincing him. The doctor diagnosed a severe case of cellulitis, and he spent a week in the hospital receiving intravenous antibiotics.

When he arrived home, he stayed sick in bed for another two weeks. Meanwhile, his business failed. Contracts stopped coming in totally, and he knew that after his guys finished their current assignments, he'd have to let them go. Teresa scheduled an appointment for him to see Dr. Randall, and he went. Randall outlined the gastric bypass surgery and informed him candidly about the hazards. There was a one-in-two hundred probability of dying and a one-in-ten likelihood of an unfavourable outcome, such as bleeding, infection, stomach ulcers, blood clots, or leakage into the belly. The doctor also warned him that it would change the way he ate permanently. Vincent Caselli, unable to work, humiliated, unwell, and in pain, determined that surgery was his only option.

It's difficult to consider human desire without asking if we have any control over our life at all. We believe in will—the idea that we have a choice in things as simple as whether to sit or stand, talk or not chat, or eat a slice of pie. However, few persons, whether heavy or thin, can maintain a voluntary weight loss for an extended period. The history of weight-loss treatment is one of almost constant failure. Regardless of the regimen—liquid diets, high-protein diets, grapefruit diets, the Zone, Atkins, or Dean Ornish diet—people lose weight quickly but do not keep it off. A 1993 National Institutes of Health expert panel examined decades of diet studies and discovered that between 90 and 95 percent of persons regained one-third to two-thirds of their lost weight within a year—and all of it within five years. Doctors have wired patients' jaws shut, inflated plastic balloons inside their stomachs, performed massive excisions of body fat, prescribed amphetamines and large amounts of thyroid hormone, and even performed neurosurgery to destroy the hunger centres in the brain's hypothalamus—and people still don't lose weight. Jaw wiring, for example, can result in significant weight loss, and patients who request the surgery are highly motivated; yet, some still consume enough liquid calories via their closed jaws to gain weight, and others regain it once the wires are withdrawn. Our species evolved to tolerate famine, not to oppose abundance.

Dinner is the moment when everything becomes clear. There are at least two ways for humans to eat more than they should at one sitting. One is to eat slowly and steadily for much too long. This is what individuals with Prader-Willi syndrome do. They have a rare hereditary hypothalamic abnormality that prevents them from experiencing satiety. And, despite eating half as quickly as most people, they do not stop. Unless their access to food is severely regulated (some will eat garbage or pet food if nothing else is available), they will become morbidly obese.

Apparently, how heavy one becomes is influenced in part by how the hypothalamus and brain stem interpret conflicting signals from the mouth and gut. Some people become full early in a meal, while others, such as Vincent Caselli, enjoy the appetiser effect for much longer. Much has been learned about the mechanisms underlying this control over the last many years. We now know, for example, that hormones such as leptin and neuropeptide Y rise and decrease in response to fat levels, adjusting hunger accordingly. However, our understanding of these systems remains limited.

Consider the 1998 report on two guys, "BR" and "RH," who suffered from extreme amnesia. They, like the protagonist in the film Memento, could hold a reasonable discussion with you, but once distracted, they remembered nothing from as recently as a minute ago, not even that they were speaking with you. (BR experienced a case of viral encephalitis, while RH had a severe seizure problem for 20 years.) Paul Rozin, a psychology professor at the University of Pennsylvania, considered employing them in an experiment to investigate the relationship between memory and food. On three consecutive days, he and his crew delivered each subject's usual meal (BR received beef loaf, barley soup, tomatoes, potatoes, beans, bread, butter, peaches, and tea; RH received veal parmigiana with pasta, string beans, juice, and apple crumb cake). Every day, BR ate his entire lunch, while RH was unable to finish. The plates were then taken away. Ten to thirty minutes later, the researchers would return with the identical meal. "Here's lunch," they would say. The males ate exactly as much as before. Another ten to thirty minutes later, the researchers returned with the same meal. "Here's lunch," they would remark, and the soldiers would continue to eat. In a few cases, the researchers offered RH a fourth lunch. Only then did he decline, citing that his "stomach was a little tight." Stomach stretch receptors were not fully ineffective. However, in the absence of a memory of having eaten, social context—someone stepping in with lunch—was sufficient to rekindle hunger.

It was 1985. Doctors were experimenting with extreme obesity surgery, but there was little enthusiasm for it. Two surgeries had shown significant promise. One procedure, known as jejuno-ileal bypass, in which nearly all of the small intestine is bypassed, allowing only a little amount of food to be digested, has been linked to death. The other, stomach stapling, was losing effectiveness over time; people adapted to the small stomach by eating heavily caloric items more frequently. However, the alterations were not limited to physical appearance. She had gradually developed a powerful and unfamiliar sensation of determination over eating. She no longer had to eat anything. "Whenever I eat somewhere along the way, I end up asking myself, 'Is this good for you? Are you going to gain weight if you eat too much of this? And I can simply stop." She couldn't understand how she felt. She realised cognitively that the surgery was why she wasn't eating as much as she used to. However, she felt as if she was choosing not to do it.

It was 1985. Doctors were experimenting with extreme obesity surgery, but there was little enthusiasm for it. Two surgeries had shown significant promise. One procedure, known as jejuno-ileal bypass, in which nearly all of the small intestine is bypassed, allowing only a little amount of food to be digested, has been linked to death. The other, stomach stapling, was losing effectiveness over time; people adapted to the small stomach by eating heavily caloric items more frequently. However, the alterations were not limited to physical appearance. She had gradually developed a powerful and unfamiliar sensation of determination over eating. She no longer had to eat anything. "Whenever I eat somewhere along the way, I end up asking myself, 'Is this good for you? Are you going to gain weight if you eat too much of this? And I can simply stop." She couldn't understand how she felt. She realised cognitively that the surgery was why she wasn't eating as much as she used to. However, she felt as if she was choosing not to do it.

It was 1985. Doctors were experimenting with extreme obesity surgery, but there was little enthusiasm for it. Two surgeries had shown significant promise. One procedure, known as jejuno-ileal bypass, in which nearly all of the small intestine is bypassed, allowing only a little amount of food to be digested, has been linked to death. The other, stomach stapling, was losing effectiveness over time; people adapted to the small stomach by eating heavily caloric items more frequently. However, the alterations were not limited to physical appearance. She had gradually developed a powerful and unfamiliar sensation of determination over eating. She no longer had to eat anything. "Whenever I eat somewhere along the way, I end up asking myself, 'Is this good for you? Are you going to gain weight if you eat too much of this? And I can simply stop." She couldn't understand how she felt. She realised cognitively that the surgery was why she wasn't eating as much as she used to. However, she felt as if she was choosing not to do it.

It took several months before I met Vince Caselli again. Winter arrived, so I called to check how he was doing. He stated he was fine, and I didn't ask for more information. When we discussed getting together, he said that it would be fun to go to a Boston Bruins game together, which piqued my interest. Perhaps he was doing fine.

A few days later, he drove me to the hospital in his booming six-wheel Dodge Ram. For the first time since I met him, he appeared practically little in that enormous truck. I inquired as to what had changed since the previous spring when I last saw him. He couldn't say exactly, but he did give me an example. "I used to love Italian cookies, and I still do," he stated. A year ago, he would have eaten till he was nauseated. "But now, I'm not sure, they're too sweet. I eat one right now, and after one or two bites, I don't want it." The same was true for pasta, which he had always struggled with. "Now I can have a taste and I'm satisfied."

Obesity surgery's success, rather than its failure, is now the source of concern. For a long period, it was considered a bastard child in reputable surgical circles. Bariatric surgeons, as obesity surgery specialists are known, faced widespread scepticism about the wisdom of proceeding with such a radical operation when so many previous versions had failed, and there was sometimes fierce opposition to even presenting their findings at the top surgical conferences. They sensed other surgeons' scorn for their patients (who were perceived to have an emotional, even moral, problem) and frequently for themselves.

It's all changed now. The American College of Surgeons recently recognized bariatric surgery as a valid specialty. The National Institutes of Health published a consensus statement recommending gastric bypass surgery as the only known effective treatment for morbid obesity, capable of producing long-term weight loss and improved health. Most insurers have agreed to pay for it. Perhaps the most frightening aspect of the growing popularity of gastric bypass surgery is the society that surrounds it. Our culture views fatness as synonymous with failure, and get-thin-quick promises, no matter how risky, can be alluring. Doctors may prescribe surgery out of concern for their patients' health, but the stigma of obesity is undoubtedly what pushes many patients to the operating room.

Indeed, electing not to have the procedure if you qualified may be judged irrational. A three-hundred-fifty-pound lady who refused the operation told me that doctors browbeat her for her decision. And I've learnt that at least one woman with heart trouble was denied care unless she underwent a gastric bypass. Some doctors persuade their patients that if they do not undergo surgery, they will die. But we don't know this. Despite significant gains in weight and health, studies have yet to demonstrate a matching reduction in death.

There are real reasons to be wary of the procedure. As Paul Ernsberger, an obesity researcher at Case Western Reserve University, pointed out to me, many gastric bypass patients are in their twenties and thirties. "But is this really going to be effective and worthwhile over a forty-year span?" wondered the man. "No one can say." He was concerned about the potential long-term consequences of dietary deficits (patients are advised to take a daily multivitamin). And he was concerned by findings from rats suggesting an increased risk of colon cancer.

We want medical advancement to be clear and unmistakable, but that rarely happens. Every new treatment involves unanswered questions—for both patients and society—and it can be difficult to decide how to address them. Perhaps a simpler, less radical procedure will be beneficial in treating obesity. Perhaps the long-awaited satiety pill will be discovered. Nonetheless, the gastric bypass is the only thing we now have that works. Although not all of the questions have been resolved, more than a decade of research has gone into it. So we forge ahead. Obesity surgery clinics are being built all around the country, and strengthened operating tables are being ordered. Surgeons and personnel are also being trained. At the same time, everyone believes that something new and better will be discovered, rendering what we are currently doing obsolete.

Part 3: Uncertainty

Chapter 11: Final Cut

You can't be mealymouthed about it anymore. I once cared for a woman in her eighties who had handed in her driver's licence only to be hit by a car driven by someone even older while walking to the bus stop. She died a few days later from a depressed skull fracture and brain haemorrhage, despite having surgery. So, on the spring afternoon that the patient gave her last breath, I stood with her and lowered my head alongside the bereaved family. Then, as politely as I could—not even saying the horrible word—I added, "If it's all right, we'd like to do an examination to confirm the cause of death."

I recently went to see the dissection of a thirty-eight-year-old woman I had cared for who had died after a long battle with heart disease. The dissecting room was located in the sub-basement, behind the laundry and loading dock, behind an unmarked metal door. It featured lofty ceilings, fading paint, and a brown tiled floor that sloped down to a central drain. A Bunsen burner was on a countertop, as was an old-style grocer's hanging scale for measuring organs, complete with a large clock-face red-arrow gauge and a pan below. Grey sections of the brain, colon, and other organs were soaking in formalin in Tupperware-style containers on shelves throughout the room. The facilities appeared rundown, chintzy, and low-tech. My patient lay on a rickety gurney in the corner, utterly naked. The autopsy team had only begun its work.

Dissections are even more gruesome than other surgical procedures. Even in the most brutal operations, such as skin grafting and amputations, surgeons maintain a sense of sensitivity and aestheticism toward their profession. We know that the bodies we cut are still alive and will awaken again. However, in the dissecting room, where the individual is gone and only the shell remains, there is little delicacy, and the difference can be seen in the slightest aspects. For example, consider how a body is transported from gurney to table. In the operation area, we use a canvas-sleeved rolling board and a series of gentle movements to transport an unconscious patient. We don't even want a bruise. Down here, by contrast, someone grabbed my patient's arm, another a leg, and simply tugged. Her skin became stuck to the stainless-steel dissecting table, so they had to moisten her and the table with a hose before pulling her the rest of the way.

Despite this, I had to concede that the patient appeared unperturbed. The assistant had followed standard practice and kept the skull incision behind the woman's ears, entirely hidden by her hair. She had also taken care to properly close the breast and abdomen by mending the wound with braided seven-cord thread. My patient appeared to be the same as previously, with the exception of a small collapse in the centre. (The normal consent form authorises the hospital to store the organs for testing and study. This popular and long-established practice has sparked outrage in Britain—the media has dubbed it "organ stripping"—but it is widely tolerated in America. Most families still do open-casket funerals following autopsies. Morticians use fillers to restore a corpse's contour, and when they're finished, you can't tell that an autopsy was performed.

Still, when it comes time to ask a family's consent to perform such a thing, the images weigh heavily on everyone's minds, including the doctor. You endeavour to maintain a cool, detached demeanour regarding these issues. But doubts do sneak in.

Even in the nineteenth century, long after religious restrictions had been relaxed, people in the West rarely allowed doctors to autopsy their loved ones for medical reasons. As a result, the practice was mostly secretive. Some doctors performed autopsies on hospital patients immediately after they died, before relatives could object. Others waited until burial and then plundered the graves, either personally or with accomplices, a practice that persisted until the twentieth century. To prevent such autopsies, some families would station nightly guards at the gravesite—hence the name "graveyard shift." Others put big stones on the coffins. In 1878, one business in Columbus, Ohio, even sold "torpedo coffins," which were outfitted with pipe bombs designed to explode if tampered with. Nonetheless, doctors remained unconvinced. In his 1906 book The Devil's Dictionary, Ambrose Bierce defined "grave" as "a place in which the dead are laid to await the coming of the medical student."

However, by the turn of the twentieth century, notable physicians such as Rudolf Virchow in Berlin, Karl Rokitansky in Vienna, and William Osler in Baltimore had gained widespread support for autopsy. They defended it as a discovery tool, noting that it has previously been used to uncover the origin of tuberculosis, reveal how to treat appendicitis, and establish Alzheimer's disease. They also demonstrated that autopsies reduced errors—without them, clinicians would not know when their diagnosis was inaccurate. Furthermore, most deaths were a mystery at the time, and perhaps what cinched the argument was the idea that autopsies could offer families with answers, giving the tale of a loved one's life a comprehensible finish.

Instead, I believe that what inhibits autopsies is medicine's arrogant, twenty-first-century attitude. I did not ask Mrs. Sykes if we might autopsy her husband because I was concerned about the cost or that the autopsy would reveal an error. The contrary was true: I didn't believe there was a good chance of finding an error. Today, we have MRI scans, ultrasounds, nuclear medicine, molecular testing, and much more. When someone dies, we know exactly why. We do not need an autopsy to find out.

Or so I thought. Then a patient changed my opinion. He was in his fifties, whiskered and jovial, a retired engineer who had found success as an artist. I'll name him Mr. Jolly since that's who he was.

Mr. Jolly had visited the hospital for treatment of a wound infection in his legs. However, he quickly developed congestive heart failure, which caused fluid to back up into his lungs. His breathing grew increasingly difficult, and we had to admit him to the intensive care unit, intubate him, and put him on a ventilator. A two-day hospitalisation evolved into two weeks. However, with a diuretic regimen and a change in heart meds, his heart failure was reversed and his lungs improved. And one sunny Sunday morning, he was relaxing in bed, breathing on his own, and watching the morning shows on the TV set suspended from the ceiling.

Two hours later, a code-blue emergency call was broadcast over the overhead speakers. When I arrived at the ICU and saw the nurse hunched over Mr. Jolly, giving chest compressions, I let out an angry curse. He'd been OK, the nurse explained, just watching TV when he abruptly sat up with a shocked expression and fell back, unconscious. He was first asystolic—no cardiac beat on the monitor—and then the rhythm returned, but there was no pulse. A swarm of employees began to work. I intubated him, administered fluids and epinephrine, had someone call the attending surgeon at home, and had another person check the morning lab test results. An X-ray technician exposed a portable chest film.

I mentally ran over the various possibilities. There weren't many. A collapsed lung, yet I heard good breath sounds with my stethoscope, and when his X-ray came back, the lungs appeared great. A significant blood loss, although his abdomen was not swollen, and his collapse occurred so swiftly that bleeding made no sense. It could have been due to extreme blood acidity, but his lab tests were normal. Then there was cardiac tamponade—bleeding into the sac that houses the heart. I loaded a six-inch spinal needle into a syringe, put it through the skin beneath the breastbone, and advanced it to the heart sac. I discovered no bleeding. That left just one possibility: a pulmonary embolism, which is a blood clot that flips into the lung and immediately blocks all blood supply. Nothing could be done about it.

I stepped out and spoke with the attending surgeon on the phone, followed by the chief resident, who had just arrived. They all agreed that an embolism was the only plausible explanation. I returned to the room and halted the code. "Time of death: 10:23 a.m.," I announced. I called his wife at home, informed her that things had gotten worse, and urged her to come in.

This should not have happened, I was certain of it. I scanned the records for clues. Then I discovered one. In a lab test the day before, the patient's clotting appeared delayed, which was not worrisome, but an ICU physician chose to treat it with vitamin K. A common negative effect of vitamin K is blood clots. I was infuriated. Giving the vitamin was absolutely unneeded; it was simply a way to manipulate a lab test result. Both the chief resident and I slammed the physician. We all but accused him of murdering the patient.

When Mrs. Jolly came, we led her to a family room that was quiet and peaceful. I could see from her expression that she had already assumed the worst. We told her that his heart had stopped suddenly due to a pulmonary embolism. We stated that the medications we gave him may have contributed to it. I brought her in to see him and left her with him. After a while, she emerged, her hands quivering and her face stained with tears. Then, unexpectedly, she thanked us. We'd kept him for her all these years, she explained. Maybe so, but neither of us felt proud of what had just happened.

I was not assigned to the operating room the next morning, so I walked down to witness the autopsy. When I arrived, Mr. Jolly was already lying on the dissecting table, his limbs splayed, skin flayed back, chest exposed, and abdomen open. I put on a gown, gloves, and a mask and approached closely. The helper started buzzing through the ribs on the left side with the electric saw, and blood began to leak out, as dark and thick as crankcase oil. Puzzled, I assisted him in opening the rib cage. The left side of the chest was filled with blood. I felt along the pulmonary arteries for a hardened, embolized clot, but found none. He hadn't had an embolism after all. We suctioned three litres of blood, lifted the left lung, and the solution emerged in front of us. The thoracic aorta was over three times its normal size, with a half-inch hole. The man had ruptured an aortic aneurysm and died nearly immediately.

In the days that followed, I apologised to the doctor for my outburst over the vitamin and wondered how we had missed the diagnosis. I examined the patient's previous X-rays and noticed a murky outline of what must have been his aneurysm. But none of us, including the radiologists, had caught it. Even if we had detected it, we would not have ventured to intervene until weeks after treating his infection and heart failure, which would have been too late. It bothered me, however, that I had been so certain about what had transpired that day and had been so mistaken.

How often do autopsies reveal a major misdiagnosis in the cause of death? I would have assumed that this occurred infrequently, perhaps in 1 or 2 percent of cases. According to three surveys conducted in 1998 and 1999, the figure is around 40%. A thorough study of autopsy studies concluded that in approximately one-third of the misdiagnoses, individuals could have survived if adequate care had been provided. George Lundberg, a pathologist and past editor of the Journal of the American Medical Association, has done more than anybody to draw attention to these statistics. He highlights the most shocking fact: the rates of misdiagnosis in autopsy investigations have not improved since at least 1938.

Chapter 12: The Dead Baby Mystery

Between 1949 and 1968, Marie Noe, a Philadelphia woman, had ten children, each of whom died. One was stillborn. One died in the hospital shortly after birth. However, eight additional newborns died at home in their cribs, where Noe reported finding them blue, limp, or gasping for air. Doctors, including some of the most respected pathologists of the period, were unable to explain the eight crib deaths, despite conducting examinations in each case. Foul play was seriously considered, but no evidence of it was discovered. Later, the medical community recognized that hundreds of seemingly healthy children died inexplicably in their beds each year, a phenomenon known as Sudden Infant Death Syndrome, or SIDS, and the cases were attributed to it.

The early SIDS notion, that newborns simply stopped breathing, has been debunked. Two intriguing findings are that sleeping on soft bedding and sleeping facedown increase a baby's chance of sudden death. An effective program to encourage parents to put their kids to bed on their backs or sides resulted in a 38 percent decrease in SIDS deaths over four years. SIDS may turn out to be a strange event in which babies, unable to turn over, are smothered by their own bedding. The findings raise doubts about how you might reliably discriminate between suffocation and SIDS—especially in the Noe instances, where the original examinations found no signs of force and the corpses were now nothing but bone. Forensic pathologists and child abuse experts I contacted verified that there is no unique postmortem finding or novel test that can distinguish SIDS from homicide by suffocation.

In child abuse trials, as in many other situations, science can only supply circumstantial evidence. True, we doctors occasionally find direct and persuasive evidence for diagnosis: burns that could only be caused by cigarettes, bruises that trace the outline of a coat hanger, and a uniform, stocking-like burn indicating a foot plunged into and held down in hot liquid. I once cared for a crying two-month-old kid whose face had been severely scalded; his father said it was the result of unintentionally turning on the hot water tap while bathing him. However, the lack of a splash pattern on the burns led the researchers to assume mistreatment. We obtained full-body X-rays of the child to look for additional damage. He had five to eight rib fractures, as well as leg fractures. Some were several weeks old. Somewhere new. Genetic and collagen testing ruled out bone and metabolic disorders that could explain such severe injuries. This was clear evidence of abuse, and the boy was taken away from his parents. Even then, as my testimony at trial showed, our evidence could not determine which of them caused the harm. (The police investigation ultimately cemented the case against the father, and a jury sentenced him to jail for felony child abuse.) Most cases do not involve such clear physical symptoms of maltreatment. When considering whether to impose the department of social services or the police on a family, we typically have only imprecise clues to go on. According to recommendations adopted at Children's Hospital in Boston, any bruise, face laceration, or long-bone fracture in an infant should be considered evidence of suspected abuse. There's not much to go on. Finally, doctors expect parents to tell us far more than physical evidence can.

A few years ago, my one-year-old daughter Hattie was playing in our playroom when she let out a gut-wrenching scream. My wife went in and discovered her lying on the ground, her right arm bent like an extra joint between the elbow and the wrist. As far as we could tell, she had attempted to climb onto our futon couch, only to have her arm trapped in the slats and then accidentally pushed over by Walker, who was two years old at the time. As she fell, her forearm bones snapped in two. When I got to the hospital with her, three separate people questioned me, repeatedly asking, "Now, exactly how did this happen?" I recognized it was a strange story—an unwitnessed fall that resulted in a severe long-bone fracture. The doctors were looking for contradictions or changes in the tale told by the parents, just as I would with any child trauma victim. It's natural for parents to feel outraged and self-righteous when doctors ask questions like cops, yet as advanced as medicine has grown, inquiries remain our primary diagnostic tool for detecting abuse.

Ultimately, I must have alleviated any fears. My daughter received a pink cast, and I took her home without incident. I couldn't help but suspect that my social standing played a factor in all of this. Even if doctors try to avoid it, social issues inevitably play a part when deciding whether to contact officials in a certain case. We know, for example, that single parents are nearly twice as likely to abuse their children as poor families. We know that one-third of crack addict mothers harm or neglect their children. (By the way, race is not a factor.) The profile is constantly in mind.

In the instance of Marie Noe, the elements worked in her favour. She was married, middle-class, and well-respected. But the fact that eight people died must imply something, right? According to one medical examiner engaged in the reopened cases, "One SIDS death is a tragedy." Two is a riddle. "Three is murder."

The real answer, however, is that, while the pattern appears to be damning enough on its own, it fails to satisfy reasonable doubts. Defying his colleagues, Pittsburgh Medical Examiner Cyril Wecht stated unequivocally that repeated SIDS deaths in one household do not necessarily imply murder. The statistics do make the Noe fatalities suspicious, he says. After all, specialists now feel that losing one infant to SIDS does not enhance the likelihood that the family will lose another. Even two fatalities in one family need scrutiny. However, Wecht went on to say that there have been situations of two or three inexplicable newborn deaths in a household where homicide was ruled out. Parents of SIDS babies have been falsely charged in the past. Worst of all, we have no idea what SIDS is. We may have combined numerous separate disorders when describing the condition. Multiple natural deaths in a family are feasible, albeit extremely unusual.

Nonetheless, while science frequently fails to show even fatal child abuse, it is not without strength. When confronted by police with medical "proof" of her homicides, Noe acknowledged suffocating four of her children and claimed she couldn't remember what happened to the others. Her lawyer quickly questioned the credibility and admissibility of the confession, which was collected after an all-night questioning. Marie Noe, on the other hand, stood up in a Philadelphia Common Pleas Court chamber on June 28, 1999, and pleaded guilty to eight charges of second-degree murder while using her cane to steady herself. Arthur, her husband of seventy-seven years, shook his head in amazement while sitting in the gallery.

Finally, what people tell us can be the most convincing evidence we have.

Chapter 13: Whose Body Is It, Anyway?

The first time I saw the patient was the day before his surgery, and I assumed he had died. Joseph Lazaroff, as I'll name him, lay in bed with his eyes closed and a cover drawn up over his tiny, birdlike chest. When people are asleep—or even when they are sedated and not breathing on their own—you don't wonder if they are still alive. They emanate life like heat. It's obvious in the tone of an arm muscle, the supply curve of their lips, and the flush on their skin. But when I bent forward to tap Lazaroff on the shoulder, I was stopped short by the natural fear of touching the deceased. His hue was all wrong—pallid and fading. His cheekbones, eyes, and temples were sunken, and his skin was stretched across his face like a mask. Strangest of all, his head was hung two inches above his pillow, as if rigour mortis had taken hold.

I was in my first year of surgical residency and was part of the neurosurgery team at the time. Lazaroff's cancer had spread throughout his body, and he was scheduled for surgery to remove a tumour from his spine. The senior resident had asked me to "consent" him—that is, to obtain Lazaroff's signature granting final authorization for the operation. "No problem," I answered. But now, looking at this fragile, withered man, I had to question if we were right to operate on him.

Then he had many nasty falls; his legs had become uncontrollably weak. He also got incontinent. He went back to see his oncologist. A scan revealed that a metastasis had compressed his thoracic spinal cord. The oncologist admitted him to the hospital and administered a round of radiation, which had no impact. Indeed, he lost the ability to move his right leg and his lower body became paralyzed. He had two choices left. He could have spinal surgery. It wouldn't cure him—surgery or not, he only had a few months left—but it did provide a last-ditch attempt to slow the course of spinal-cord injury and potentially restore some strength to his legs and sphincters. The hazards, however, were considerable. We'd have to enter through his chest and burst his lung merely to get to his spine. He would have a lengthy, tough, and painful recovery. And, given his poor health and previous history of heart illness, his odds of surviving the procedure and returning home were slim.

Jay Katz, a Yale doctor and ethicist, wrote a book in 1984 called The Silent World of Doctor and Patient, which contributed to this drastic shift in how medical decisions are made. It was a stinging critique of traditional medical decision-making, and it had a broad impact. Katz claimed in the book that patients have the ability and responsibility to make medical decisions. And he used actual patient anecdotes to make his case. One was that of "Iphigenia Jones," a twenty-one-year-old lady who was diagnosed with cancer in one of her breasts. She had two alternatives back then, as she has now: mastectomy (removal of the breast and adjacent axillary lymph nodes) or radiation with minimum surgery (removal of only the lump and lymph nodes). Survival rates were comparable, however in a spared breast, the tumour can reappear and necessitate surgery. This surgeon preferred to perform mastectomies, and he informed her that was what he would do. However, in the days preceding the operation, the surgeon became concerned about removing someone's breast at such a young age. So the night before the operation, he did something unusual: he discussed the therapy choices with her and let her decide. She chose breast-conserving therapy.

Medical schools eventually agreed with Katz's position. By the early 1990s, we had been indoctrinated to view patients as autonomous decision makers. "You work for them," I was repeatedly reminded. Many old-school doctors continue to try to dictate from on high, but patients are no longer willing to tolerate it. Most doctors, who believe that patients should have authority over their own lives, explain the options and hazards. Some even refuse to give advice for fear of negatively influencing patients. Patients ask questions, look up information online, and seek second viewpoints. They make a decision.

In actuality, however, things aren't as simple. Patients, it turns out, make poor decisions too. Of course, there are situations when the difference between two options is insignificant.

Lazaroff sought surgery. The oncologist was unsure about the decision, so she consulted a neurosurgeon. The neurosurgeon, a trim man in his forties with a superb reputation and a penchant for bow ties, met Lazaroff and his kid that afternoon. He warned them repeatedly about the grave risks and the limited potential return. Sometimes, he explained later, people don't appear to hear the concerns, and in those circumstances, he is especially emphatic about them—being stuck on a ventilator due to poor lung function, having a stroke, dying. But Lazaroff was not to be deterred. The surgeon added him to the schedule.

Lazaroff underwent surgery the next day. After undergoing anaesthesia, he was rolled onto his left side. A thoracic surgeon created a deep incision into the chest cavity from the front to the back along the eighth rib, inserted a rib spreader, cranked it open, and secured a retractor to keep the deflated lung out of the way. You could see clear down the back of the chest to the spinal column. A meaty, tennis ball-sized tumour engulfed the eleventh vertebra. The neurosurgeon took over and performed a thorough dissection around and beneath the tumour. It took a few hours, but the tumour was finally connected just where it had infiltrated the bone vertebral body. He then used a rongeur—a hard, jawed instrument—to make little, meticulous bites in the vertebral body, similar to a beaver nibbling steadily through a tree trunk, eventually removing the vertebra and, with it, the lump. To rebuild the spine, he filled the remaining gap with a doughy plug of methacrylate, an acrylic cement, and allowed it to set over time. He inserted a probe behind the new artificial vertebrae. There was ample space. It took more than four hours, but the pressure on the spinal cord was relieved. The thoracic surgeon closed Lazaroff's chest, leaving a rubber chest tube protruding to reinflate his lung, and he was taken to critical care.

The procedure was technically successful. Lazaroff's lungs did not recover, and we struggled to get him off the ventilator. Over the next three days, they stiffened and became fibrotic, necessitating higher ventilator pressures. We tried to keep him sedated, but he frequently broke free and awoke wild-eyed and thrashing.

The neurosurgeon approached me with the news. I walked to Lazaroff's ICU room, which was one of eight bays arranged in a semicircle around a nursing station, each with a tile floor, a window, and a sliding glass door that kept the noise out but not the nurses' gaze. A nurse and I slipped inside. I double-checked that Lazaroff's morphine drip was set to the maximum level. I took my place at his bedside, leaned in close to him, and told him, in case he could hear me, that I was about to remove the breathing tube from his mouth. I removed the tube's ties and deflated the balloon cuff that held it in his trachea. Then I took the tube out. He coughed several times, opened his eyes briefly, and then closed them. The nurse suctioned the mucus from his mouth. I turned off the ventilator, and the room became quiet except for the sound of his laborious, gasping gasps. We watched him tire out. His breathing slowed until he could only take short, agonising gasps before coming to a halt. I placed my stethoscope on his chest and listened as his heart faded away. Thirteen minutes after I pulled him off the ventilator, I instructed the nurse to document Joseph Lazaroff's death.

I think Lazaroff made a horrible decision. Not, however, because he died so violently and horribly. Good judgments can have negative consequences (occasionally people must take awful risks), and bad decisions can have positive consequences ("Better luck than good," surgeons say). I think Lazaroff made a horrible decision because it went against his innermost interests—not as I or anybody else conceived them, but as he conceived them. Above all, he clearly wanted to live. He would take any danger, including death, to live. However, as we explained to him, life was not something we had to provide. We could only offer him a chance of keeping minimal lower-body function for his brief remaining time, at the expense of great violence and the risk of a terrible death. But he didn't hear us: he appeared to assume that by avoiding paralysis, he could avoid death. Some folks will look at the odds and decide to go forward with surgery. But, knowing how much Lazaroff hated dying like his wife had, I don't think he was one of them.

I had entered residency to study how to be a surgeon. I had assumed that meant just knowing the repertoire of motions and procedures used in performing a surgery or making a diagnosis. In reality, there was also the new and sensitive task of guiding patients through their decisions, which sometimes required its own set of manoeuvres and procedures.

Suppose you're a doctor. You're in your clinic's examination room—one of those tiny spaces with fluorescent lights, a Matisse picture on the wall, a box of latex gloves on the counter, and a cold, padded patient table as the centrepiece—to see a female patient in her forties. She is a mother of two and a partner at a downtown law company. Despite the circumstances and her flimsy paper gown, she maintains her cool. You detect no lumps or abnormalities in her breasts. She underwent a mammography before visiting you, and you are now reviewing the radiologist's report, which states, "There is a faint group of punctate, clustered calcifications in the upper outer quadrant of the left breast that were not clearly present on the prior examination." A biopsy must be performed to rule out the risk of cancer." Translation: concerning features have emerged; they could indicate breast cancer.

However, these calcifications are not ambiguous observations. They frequently signify cancer—even if not always—and are usually detected at an early and treatable stage. If having power over one's life means anything, people must be allowed to make their own errors. However, when the stakes are this high and a mistake decision could be irrevocable, doctors are hesitant to sit back. This is when they typically push. So, push. Your patient is about to walk out the door. You might halt her in her tracks and inform her that she is making a terrible mistake. Give her a lengthy lecture about cancer. Point out the folly of assuming that three negative biopsies mean that the fourth will be negative as well. In all likelihood, you'll lose her. The goal is not to demonstrate to her how mistaken she is. The goal is to offer her the opportunity to change her mind.

And so, when the team of doctors arrived to discuss whether to intubate Hunter, I wanted them to make the decision—doctors I had never met before. Jay Katz, an ethicist, and others have criticised this type of desire as "childlike regression." But that judgement appears heartless to me. The uncertainties were brutal, and I couldn't face the thought of making the incorrect decision. Even if I was confident that I had made the best decision for her, I couldn't bear the guilt if something went wrong. Some feel that patients should be urged to take responsibility for their decisions. However, that would have appeared to be harsh paternalism in its own right. I needed Hunter's physicians to take responsibility: they could deal with the repercussions, good or bad.

I delegated decision-making authority to the doctors, who made it immediately. They told me they'd keep Hunter off the ventilator. And with that, the bleary-eyed, stethoscope-wearing group trudged on to their next patient. Still, there was the lingering question: if I wanted to make the best decision for Hunter, was giving up my hard-earned liberty truly the right thing to do? Carl Schneider, a professor of law and medicine at the University of Michigan, recently published The Practice of Autonomy, in which he sifted through a plethora of studies and data on medical decision making, including a thorough review of patients' memoirs. He discovered that the ill were frequently unable to make sound decisions because they were weary, irritated, devastated, or depressed. They were often too preoccupied with their immediate discomfort, nausea, and weariness to consider important decisions. This rang true for me. I wasn't even the patient, so all I could do was sit and watch Hunter, worry, or distract myself with busywork. I didn't have the focus or energy to adequately weigh the therapeutic alternatives.

Being a patient is an art form in the same way that being a doctor is. You must make sensible decisions about whether to acquiesce and when to express yourself. Even if a patient chooses not to make a decision, they should challenge their doctors and demand explanations. I may have allowed Hunter's physicians to take control, but I insisted on a clear strategy in case she crashed. Later, I became concerned that they were feeding her too slowly—she hadn't eaten anything in over a week, and I pestered them with inquiries about why. When they pulled her off the oxygen monitor on her eleventh day in the hospital, I became concerned. What was the harm in keeping it on? I inquired. I'm sure I was stubborn, even wrongheaded, at times. You do your best, taking into account your doctors and nurses as well as your personal position, trying not to be too passive or pushy for your own good.

Several ethicists make the mistake of emphasising patient autonomy as the ultimate ideal in medicine, rather than acknowledging it as one among several. Schneider discovered that what patients want most from doctors is competence and kindness, rather than autonomy. Now, kindness often entails respecting patients' autonomy and ensuring that they have influence over critical decisions. However, it may also entail making difficult decisions when patients do not want to, or leading them in the correct way when they do. Even when patients want to make their own decisions, there are instances when it is compassionate to press them: to persuade them to undergo an operation or therapy they are afraid of, or to forgo one on which they have placed their expectations. Many ethicists find this line of thinking troubling, and medicine will continue to grapple with how patients and doctors should make choices. However, as the sector becomes more sophisticated and technological, the actual aim is not to eliminate paternalism; rather, it is to sustain kindness.

Chapter 14: The Case of the Red Leg

While seeing patients with one of the surgical professors in his clinic one afternoon, I was surprised by how frequently he had to respond to his patients' questions with, "I do not know." These are four small words that doctors are often reluctant to say. We are meant to have the solutions. We want to know the answers. But he had to say those four small words to everyone that day.

That weekend, she returned home to Hartford, Connecticut, to attend a wedding. (She had relocated to Boston with some girlfriends the year before, after graduating from Ithaca College, and found work managing conferences for a downtown law company.) The wedding had been spectacular, and she had kicked off her shoes and danced all night. However, the next morning she awoke with a hurting left foot. She had a week-old blister on the top of her foot from some cheap sandals she had worn, and the skin around it was red and puffy. She didn't think much about it at first. When she showed her father her foot, he stated it looked like a bee sting or like she had been stepped on while dancing the night before. By late afternoon, while going back to Boston with her lover, "my foot really began killing me," she admitted. The redness spread overnight, and she developed chills, sweats, and a temperature of 103 degrees. She took ibuprofen every several hours, which reduced her temperature but did nothing to alleviate the increasing pain. By morning, the redness had spread halfway up her calf, and her foot had swollen to the point where it could hardly fit into a sneaker.

Eleanor staggered in on her roommate's shoulder to visit her physician that afternoon, where she was diagnosed with cellulitis. Cellulitis is a common skin infection caused by perfectly ordinary bacteria in the environment penetrating your skin's barrier (by a cut, puncture wound, blister, or whatever) and growing within it. Eleanor discovered that your skin gets red, hot, bloated, and painful; you feel unwell; fevers are prevalent; and the infection spreads quickly along your skin. The doctor obtained an X-ray to ensure that the bone underlying was not diseased. She gave Eleanor a dose of intravenous antibiotics in the office, a tetanus shot, and a prescription for a week's worth of antibiotic pills. The doctor emphasised that while this was generally effective treatment for cellulitis, it was not always the case. She traced the red border on Eleanor's calf with an indelible black marker. If the redness spreads beyond this line, the doctor advised her to call. Regardless, she should return the next day to have the infection checked.

Eleanor reported that the next morning—this morning—she awoke with a rash beyond the black line, a piece stretching to her leg, and the discomfort was worse than before. She called the doctor, who told her to go to the ER. The doctor stated that she would need to be admitted to the hospital for a full course of intravenous antibiotics. I inquired whether Eleanor had any pus or leakage from her leg. No. Are there any sores on her skin? No. A bad odour or darkening of her skin? No. Any more fevers? No, not since two days ago. I let the information float around in my thoughts. Everything seemed to point to cellulitis. But something was pricking at me, keeping me aware.

I asked Eleanor if I could see the rashes. She pulled back the sheet. The right leg appeared to be in good condition. The left leg was red—a meaty, consistent, angry red—from her forefoot, up her ankle, up her calf, past the black ink line from the day before, to her knee, with another tongue of crimson continuing to the inner of her thigh. The border was sharp. The skin felt heated and delicate to the touch. The blister on the top of her foot was small. The skin around it had been damaged slightly. Her toes were unconcerned, and she wiggled them for me with ease. She had a tougher problem moving the foot because it was thick with edema up to the ankle. She experienced normal sensations and pulses throughout her leg. She didn't have any ulcers or pus.

Decisions in medicine are meant to be based on concrete observations and hard evidence. But only a few weeks previously, I had cared for a patient whose memory would never leave me. He was a healthy fifty-eight-year-old guy who had experienced three or four days of increasing agony on the left side of his chest, beneath his arm, where he had a fall abrasion. (To maintain confidentiality, some identifying information has been modified.) He visited a community hospital near his home to have it checked out. He was diagnosed with a minor skin rash on his chest and was given antibiotics for cellulitis before being discharged. That night, the rash had expanded eight inches. The following morning, he developed a fever of 102 degrees. By the time he returned to the emergency hospital, the affected skin had become numb and blistered. He quickly went into shock. He was taken to my hospital, and we swiftly took him to the operating room.

He didn't have cellulitis; instead, he had necrotizing fasciitis, a rare and fatal condition. It has been referred to as a disease of "flesh-eating bacteria" in the tabloids, and the word is not overblown. Opening the skin revealed a large illness that was significantly worse than what appeared on the outside. All of the muscles on the left side of his chest, from his back to his shoulder and down to his abdomen, had gone grey, mushy, and nasty from invading germs and needed to be removed. That first day in the OR, we had to remove even the muscles between his ribs, a procedure known as a birdcage thoracotomy. The following day, we had to remove his arm. For a while, we believed we had saved him. His fevers subsided, and plastic surgeons repaired his chest and abdominal wall using muscle transfers and Gore Tex sheets. However, one by one, his kidneys, lungs, liver, and heart failed, and he died. It was one of the worst cases I've ever been engaged in.

What we know about necrotizing fasciitis is that it is extremely aggressive and quickly spreads. It kills up to 70% of those who contract it. No known antibiotic can halt it. The most common bacteria implicated is group A Streptococcus (in fact, the final cultures from our patient's tissue grew exactly like this). It is a creature that typically causes nothing more than a strep throat, but some strains have evolved the ability to do far more. Nobody knows where these strains came from. They are thought to enter the body through skin breaks, similar to how cellulitis does. The break can be as significant as a surgical incision or as minor as an abrasion. (The disease has been linked to rug burns, bug bites, friendly punches in the arm, paper cuts, blood draws, toothpick injuries, and chicken pox lesions. In many cases, the entry point is never located at all. Unlike cellulitis, the bacteria enter not only the skin but also deep beneath it, rapidly moving along the outer sheaths of muscle (the fascia) and eating any soft tissue (fat, muscle, nerves, connective tissue) they come across. Survival is only possible with early and radical excisional surgery, which often necessitates amputation. To be successful, it must be completed as soon as possible. By the time indicators of deep invasion become apparent—such as shock, loss of sensation, and widespread blistering of the skin—the person is usually irreversibly damaged.

Standing at Eleanor's bedside, bent over scrutinising her leg, I felt silly given the diagnosis—it was as if the ebola virus had come into the emergency room. True, in its early stages, necrotizing fasciitis can resemble cellulitis, with the same redness, swelling, fever, and elevated white blood cell count. But there's an old adage in medical school: if you hear hoofbeats in Texas, think horses, not zebras. Each year, only approximately a thousand instances of necrotizing fasciitis are reported in the United States, primarily among the elderly and chronically ill, while more than three million cases of cellulitis are reported. Furthermore, Eleanor's fever had subsided; she did not appear abnormally ill, and I realised I was being misled by a single, recent anecdote. If there had been an easy test to distinguish between the two diagnoses, that would have been one thing. However, there is none. The only option is to go to the operating room, open the skin, and look—not something you want to suggest haphazardly.

As I hung up the phone, Eleanor's father, a brown-and-grey-haired man in his fifties, approached with a sandwich and Coke for daughter. He had been with her all day, having travelled over from Hartford, but when I saw her, he had left to get her lunch. I jumped to advise him not to let her eat or drink "just yet" when I saw the food, and the cat began creeping out of the bag. It was not an ideal approach to introduce myself. He was taken aback, realising that an empty stomach is what we require for patients going into surgery. I attempted to defuse the situation by explaining that the delay was simply "routine procedure" until we had completed our evaluation. Nonetheless, Eleanor and her father were filled with dread as Studdert appeared in his scrubs and operating hat to see her.

He asked her to repeat her narrative before uncovering her leg to examine it. He didn't appear that impressed. When we were alone, he told me that the rash looked "like a bad cellulitis." But could he be sure it wasn't necrotizing fasciitis? He couldn't. It is a fact of medicine that deciding not to do something—not ordering a test, not providing an antibiotic, or not transporting a patient to the operating room—is far more difficult than choosing to do it. Once a possibility is considered, especially one as horrific as necrotizing fasciitis, it is difficult to dismiss.

Studdert perched on the side of her bed. He told Eleanor and her father that her tale, symptoms, and exam all pointed to cellulitis, which was the most likely diagnosis. However, there was another, extremely uncommon possibility, and he went on to discuss the unquiet and ungentle effects of necrotizing fasciitis in a quiet and gentle tone. He described the "flesh-eating bacteria," the alarmingly high fatality rate, and the inability to be treated with antibiotics alone. "I think it is unlikely you have it," he said Eleanor. "I'd put the chances"—he was guessing here—"at well under five percent."

However, he said that "we cannot rule it out without a biopsy." He paused for a bit to allow her and her father to process this. Then he began to explain the process, describing how he would remove an inch or so of skin and underlying tissue from the top of her foot, and possibly from higher up on her leg, and immediately have a pathologist examine the samples under a microscope.

Eleanor became rigid. "This is crazy," she exclaimed. "This doesn't make any sense." She looked panicked, as if she were drowning. "Why don't we just wait and see how the antibiotics go?" Studdert said that this was a sickness that could not be ignored, and that in order to treat it, it had to be detected early on. Eleanor simply shook her head and glanced down at her covers.

Studdert and I both looked to her father to see what he may say. He had been silent up until this moment, standing beside her, his forehead wrinkled, hands gripped behind him, stiff, like a guy attempting to stay upright on a rocking boat. He inquired about specifics—how long a biopsy would take (fifteen minutes), what the hazards were (a deep wound infection was the most serious, oddly), whether the scars would fade (no), and when it would be completed (within an hour). He inquired cautiously about what would happen if the biopsy revealed the disease. Studdert reiterated that he believed the chances were fewer than five percent. But if she got it, he warned, we'd need to "remove all the infected tissue." He hesitated before continuing. "This could mean an amputation," he explained. Eleanor started to cry. "I don't want to do this, Dad." Mr. Bratton swallowed hard, his gaze fixated somewhere far beyond us.

In recent years, we in medicine have found how often we fail to do right by our patients. For starters, even when we know what the proper thing to do is, we often fail to execute it. Plain old execution errors are not uncommon, and we have barely begun to detect the systemic flaws, technology flaws, and human shortcomings that cause them, let alone how to mitigate them. Furthermore, vital knowledge has not been widely applied. For example, among patients who have been diagnosed with a heart attack, it is now known that taking an aspirin alone can save lives, and that using a thrombolytic—a clot-dissolving drug—right away can save even more. However, one-quarter of individuals who should receive aspirin do not, and half of those who should have thrombolytics do not. Overall, physician adherence to various evidence-based guidelines varies from more than 80% of patients in some parts of the country to fewer than 20% elsewhere. Much of medicine still lacks basic organisation and commitment to ensuring that we do what we know we should do.

However, spend any amount of time with doctors and patients, and you will discover that the larger, starker, and more unpleasant challenge is the ongoing doubt about what should be done in many circumstances. The grey zones in medicine are vast, and we are confronted with scenarios like Eleanor's on a daily basis—situations in which strong scientific evidence of what to do is lacking but decisions must be made. For example, which pneumonia patients should be admitted to the hospital and which should be discharged home? Which back symptoms are addressed surgically, and which with conservative methods alone? who patients with a rash underwent surgery, and who were simply watched on antibiotics? In many cases, the answers are obvious. However, we have no idea what happens to countless others. Expert panels tasked with reviewing actual medical decisions discovered that in a quarter of hysterectomy cases, a third of operations to insert tubes into children's ears, and a third of pacemaker insertions (to name a few examples), there was insufficient science to determine whether the procedures would benefit those specific patients.

In the lack of algorithms and data regarding what to do, medical students learn to make decisions based on their feelings. You rely on your experience and judgement. And it is difficult not to be concerned by this.

A few weeks before seeing Eleanor, I saw an arthritic and quite elderly woman (she was born before Woodrow Wilson was president) who complained of severe abdominal discomfort that spread to her back. When I learnt that she had recently been diagnosed with an abdominal aortic aneurysm, my alarm bells went out. Examining her carefully, I could feel the aneurysm, a throbbing and painful mass right beneath her abdominal muscles. She was steady, but it was on the edge of rupturing, I was certain. The vascular surgeon I phoned concurred. We informed the woman that emergency surgery was the only way to rescue her. We cautioned her, however, that it was a major surgery with a lengthy recovery in intensive care and likely in a nursing home afterward (she still lived independently), a significant danger that her kidneys would fail, and a minimum 10 to 20 percent likelihood of mortality. She didn't know what to do. We left her with her family to consider the decision, and I returned fifteen minutes later. She stated that she would not go ahead with surgery. She only wanted to go home. She has lived a long life, she explained. Her health had long been declining. She had drafted her will and was now measuring her remaining days in coffee spoons. Her family was distraught, yet she maintained a calm and steady voice. I wrote up a pain medication prescription for her son to fill, and she left half an hour later, well aware that she was going to die. I retained her son's phone number and, after a few weeks, called him at home to see how he was handling the fallout. His mother, however, answered the phone herself. I said hi and inquired how she was doing. She was doing fine and thanked you. A year later, I discovered she was still alive and living on her own.

Three decades of neuropsychology study have revealed various ways in which human judgement, like memory and hearing, is subject to systematic errors. The mind overestimates vivid risks, gets stuck in ruts, and struggles to manage large amounts of data. It is overly influenced by desire, emotion, and even the time of day. It is influenced by the order in which information is delivered and how problems are defined. And if we doctors thought that with all of our training and expertise, we were immune to such flaws, we were proven wrong when researchers examined us.

Several investigations have found that physician judgement is distorted in the same way. One study from the Medical College of Virginia discovered that doctors ordering blood cultures for patients with fever underestimated the likelihood of infection by four to ten times. Furthermore, clinicians who had recently encountered other patients with blood infections had the largest overestimates. Another study from the University of Wisconsin discovered evidence of a Lake Wobegon effect ("Lake Wobegon: where the women are strong, the men are good-looking, and all the children are above average"), in which the vast majority of surgeons believed their own patients' mortality rates were lower than the average. A study by Ohio University and Case Western Reserve Medical School looked at not only the accuracy but also the confidence of physicians' judgments—and found no link between the two. Doctors who were confident in their judgement proved to be no more accurate than doctors who were not.

In truth, there is another way to make decisions, one promoted by a small and struggling medical coterie. Decision analysis is a technique that has been employed in industry and the military for many years, and its fundamentals are basic. A decision tree is created on a piece of paper (or a computer) by listing all of your options and the probable outcomes of those selections. You calculate the chance of each occurrence numerically, using hard facts where available and a rough forecast when not. You evaluate each outcome in terms of its relative desirability (or "utility") to the patient. Then you multiply the values for each choice and select the one with the highest calculated "expected utility." The idea is to employ explicit, rational, statistical thinking rather than your gut instincts. The decision to prescribe annual mammograms for all women over the age of fifty was taken in this manner, as was the United States' choice to bail out Mexico when its economy collapsed. Why not, the advocates argue, individual patient decisions?

I recently attempted "treeing out" (as decision buffs call it) the option Eleanor faced. The choice was simple: biopsy or not biopsy. However, the outcomes immediately became convoluted. There was not being biopsied and doing fine; not being biopsied, getting diagnosed late, going through surgery, and surviving anyway; not being biopsied and dying; being biopsied and getting only a scar; being biopsied and getting a scar plus bleeding from it; being biopsied, having the disease and an amputation, but dying anyway; and so on. When all of the options and implications were mapped out, my decision tree resembled a bush. Assigning probability to each possible twist of fate appeared questionable. I gathered as much information as possible from the medical literature and then had to make significant extrapolations. Even after discussing the outcomes with Eleanor, it appeared hard to determine their relative attractiveness. Is dying a hundred times worse than doing well, a thousand times worse, or a million? Where does a scar that is bleeding fit in? Nonetheless, these are the most important elements, according to decision experts, and when we make decisions based on instinct, we are merely masking the truth.

However, producing a formal analysis within a reasonable time range proved impossible. It took a few days—not the minutes we had anticipated—and a lot of back and forth with two decision makers. But it did give an answer. According to the final decision tree, we shouldn't have gone to the operating room for a biopsy. The odds of my initial guess being correct was too low, and the probability that discovering the condition early would make no difference was too high. The argument suggested that a biopsy could not be justified.

Eleanor was put to sleep by the anesthesiologist. A nurse then painted her leg with antiseptic from the toes to the hip. Studdert used a small knife to remove an inch-long ellipse of skin and tissue from the blister on the top of her foot down to her tendon. The specimen was placed in a jar of sterile saline and promptly delivered to the pathologist for examination. We then extracted a second specimen, this time deeper into muscle, from the centre of the redness in her leg, and sent it on as well.

At first sight, there was nothing obvious beneath her skin to worry us. The fat layer was yellow, as it should be, and the muscle was a healthy gleaming red that bled properly. When we probed with the tip of a clamp inside the calf incision, it moved strangely readily along the muscle, as if bacteria had paved the way. This is not a definitive finding, but it was significant enough that Studdert exclaimed, "Oh shit." He removed his gloves and gown to see what the pathologist had discovered, and I followed right behind him, leaving Eleanor asleep in the OR to be monitored by another resident and the anesthesiologist.

A frozen section is an urgent pathology examination, and the place for it was just a few doors down the hall. The room was small, roughly the size of a kitchen. In the centre was a waist-high laboratory table with a black slate surface and a canister of liquid nitrogen, which the pathologist had used to quickly freeze the tissue samples. Along one wall was the microtome, which he had used to cut micron-thin slices of tissue to place on glass slides. We stepped in right as he finished preparing the slides. He brought them to a microscope and began scanning each one systematically, first under low power magnification and then at high power. We hovered, no likely annoyingly, waiting for the diagnosis. Minutes passed in stillness.

Studdert went to visit Eleanor's father. When he came into the busy family waiting area, Bratton noticed the expression on his face and said, "Don't look at me like that!" Do not stare at me like that!" Studdert led him into a secret side room, locked the door behind them, and informed him that she appeared to have the disease. He would need to move quickly, he said. He wasn't sure he could save her limb, or her life. He'd need to open up her leg, assess the situation, and then proceed from there. Bratton was overtaken, crying and struggling to speak. Studdert's eyes were damp. Bratton responded, "Do what you have to do." Studdert nodded and walked away. Bratton then phoned his wife. He informed her of the news and then gave her a chance to respond. "I will never forget what I heard on the other end of the line," he recalled later. "Something, some sound, I cannot and will never be able to describe."

In medicine, as in other fields, decisions compound themselves. You've hardly gotten beyond one fork in the road before another appears. The key question now was what to do. Segal joined Studdert in the operating room to provide more assistance. They split Eleanor's leg from the base of her toes, across her ankle, and just below her knee to get a good look inside. They used retractors to widen the aperture.

The sickness was clearly obvious now. Her foot and much of her calf had a grey and dead outer fascial layer of muscles. A brownish dishwater fluid was pouring out, accompanied by a faint scent of rotting. (Tissue samples and bacterial cultures eventually revealed that this was a toxic group A Streptococcus progressing fast up her leg.).

He and Segal used scissors and electrocautery for two hours to cut and strip off the necrotic outer layers of her muscle, beginning with the webbing of her toes and progressing to the tendons of her leg. They removed tissue approximately three-quarters of the way around. Her skin hung off her leg like gaping coat flaps. Higher up, inside the leg, they saw fascia that appeared pink-white, fresh, and very lively. They injected two litres of sterile saline through the leg, hoping to remove as much bacteria as possible.

Eleanor appeared to be holding solid toward the conclusion. Her blood pressure stays normal. Her temperature was ninety-nine degrees. Her oxygen levels were normal. The worst-looking tissue has been removed from her leg.

Studdert stayed solid in his decision not to take any more, but you could tell he was uneasy. He and Segal discussed another option: an experimental technique known as hyperbaric oxygen. It entailed putting Eleanor in one of those pressure chambers that divers use when they get the bends—a strange-sounding but not absurd idea. Immune cells require oxygen to properly destroy bacteria, and exposing a person to double or higher atmospheric pressure for a few hours every day significantly increases the oxygen content in tissue. Segal was impressed by the results he had obtained with the therapy in a couple of burn patients with severe wound infections. True, research had not shown that it would be effective against necrotizing fasciitis. But suppose it could? Everyone instantly accepted the treatment. At the very least, it made us feel like we were doing something to combat the infection we were leaving behind.

We didn't have a chamber at our hospital, but another one across town had. Someone picked up the phone, and within a few minutes, we had a plan in place to transport Eleanor over with one of our nurses for two hours under 2.5 atmospheres of pressure oxygen. We kept her wound open to drain, inserted wet gauze to protect the tissues from drying out, and bandaged her leg in white bandages. We wheeled her from the operating room to intensive care to ensure she was stable enough to travel.

It was now 8 p.m. Eleanor awoke feeling sick and in pain. But she was astute enough to deduce from the mass of nurses and physicians around her that something was awry.

She reached down to find it, and for a few anxious moments, she wasn't sure she could. She slowly convinced herself that she could see, touch, feel, and move it. Studdert placed his hand on her arm. He explained what he had discovered, what he had done, and what else there would be to do. She handled the knowledge with more tenacity and determination than I realised she possessed. Her entire family had arrived to be with her, and it appeared like they had been hit by an SUV. But Eleanor put the sheet back over her leg, looked at the monitors flashing green and orange lights and the IV lines flowing into her arms, and simply said, "OK."

The hyperbaric chamber that night was, as she describes it, "like a glass coffin." She lay inside on a narrow mattress with nowhere to put her arms except straight down or folded across her chest, a thick plexiglass panel a foot from her face, and an overhead hatch sealed tight with turns of a heavy wheel. As the pressure mounted, her ears continued to explode, as if she were diving into a deep ocean. The doctors had warned her that if the pressure reached a certain level, she would be stuck. Even if she started throwing up, they couldn't get to her since the pressure had only been released gradually or she'd have the bends and die. "One person had a seizure inside," she recalls them telling her. "It took them twenty minutes to get to him." Lying there imprisoned, more ill than she'd ever dreamed possible, she felt distant and almost completely alone. "It's just me and the bacteria in here," she thought to herself.

The next morning, we returned her to the operating room to determine whether the germs had spread. They had. The flesh covering the majority of her foot and the front of her leg was gangrenous and black, and it had to be removed. The borders of fascia we had left behind were dead and needed to be removed as well. Her muscles, however, remained functional, especially in her foot. And the bacteria hadn't killed anything in her thigh. She experienced no additional fevers. Her heart rate had stabilised. We repacked the wound with wet gauze and sent her back for more hyperbaric oxygen—two hours twice a day.

We wound up operating on her leg four times in four days. We had to take a bit more tissue with each procedure, but it got progressively smaller. At the third procedure, we discovered that the redness on her skin had finally begun to fade. At the fourth operation, the redness had subsided, and we could see the pink mossy beginnings of new tissue in the mouth of the incision. Studdert was only then convinced that Eleanor, as well as her foot and leg, had survived.

We don't know what to do with intuition when it works well. Such achievements are not just the outcome of logical thought. However, they are not the consequence of pure luck. Gary Klein, a cognitive psychologist who has spent his career observing people who are constantly confronted with ambiguity, recalls the story of a fire commander he once examined. The lieutenant and his squad had arrived to fight an ordinary-looking fire in a one-story house. He led the water team in from the front and came across the fire in the back kitchen area. They attempted to douse it with water. However, the flames returned. They tried sprinkling the flames again but had no effect. The crew took a few steps back to plot another line of assault. The lieutenant then abruptly ordered his men to leave the building, much to their surprise. Something didn't feel right, and he had no idea what it was. And as soon as they left, the floor they were standing on fell. The fire was found to be in the basement rather than the back. If they had lingered just a few seconds longer, they would have fallen into the fire themselves.

Sometimes humans can just recognize the proper thing to do. Klein points out that judgement is rarely a reasoned weighing of all choices, which we aren't particularly good at, but rather an unconscious form of pattern recognition. Following the incident, the commander told Klein that he had not considered the various possibilities in that residence. He still had no notion why he had gotten his guys out of there. The fire had been challenging, but not to the point that he had fled previously. The only possible explanations seemed to be luck or ESP. However, when Klein questioned him about the scene's circumstances, he discovered two signs that the lieutenant had picked up without recognizing it. The living room had been warm—warmer than he had expected from a controlled fire in the back of a house. And the fire was silent, which surprised him because he anticipated it to be noisy. The lieutenant's thinking appears to have seen a dangerous pattern in these and maybe other clues, prompting him to issue the all-out order. In fact, thinking too hard about the situation could have negated the benefit of his intuition.

It is still unclear to me what clues I was registering when I first saw Eleanor's leg. Similarly, it is unclear what symptoms indicated that we could get by without an amputation. However, as arbitrary as our intuitions appear, there must have been some underlying logic to them. What makes no sense is how anyone could have known that, or how anyone can accurately judge if a doctor's intuitions are on track or wildly wrong.

For nearly thirty years, Dartmouth physician Jack Wennberg has examined medical decision making, not up close as Gary Klein has, but from as high a vantage point as possible, looking at all American doctors. And he has discovered a tenacious, overwhelming, and embarrassing level of inconsistency in what we do. His research has revealed, for example, that the likelihood of a doctor sending you for a gallbladder removal procedure changes 270 percent depending on where you reside; for a hip replacement, 450 percent; and for care in an intensive care unit during the last six months of your life, 880 percent. A patient in Santa Barbara, California, is five times more likely to be advised to undergo back surgery for back pain than one in the Bronx, New York. This is mostly an issue of ambiguity at work, with each doctors' diverse experience, habits, and intuitions resulting in vastly different patient care.

People have presented two ways for change. One goal is to reduce uncertainty in medicine by conducting research on minor but essential everyday decisions made by patients and doctors (which now receives embarrassingly little funding). Everyone recognizes, however, that a significant deal of uncertainty about what to do for people will always exist. (Human disease and lives are too complicated for reality to be otherwise.) As a result, it has been argued, not unreasonably, that doctors must agree in advance on what should be done in uncertain situations that arise—spell out our actions ahead of time to eliminate guesswork and gain the benefit of group decision.

However, this last one goes almost nowhere. For it contradicts all that doctors believe about ourselves as persons, about our ability to reason with patients about what is best for them. In all of the uncertainty caused by the various techniques that different doctors take to a given problem, someone must get it right. And each of us, who are accustomed to make judgments in the face of uncertainty on a daily basis, believes that someone is me. For as many times our judgement fails us, we all have Eleanor Bratton, our great improbable saving.

It was a year before I saw Eleanor again. While passing through Hartford, I stopped by her family's home, a large, spic-and-span, putty-colored colonial with a galumphy dog and flower beds outside. Eleanor had returned home to recover after spending twelve days in the hospital, expecting to stay only temporarily but finding herself settling in. She admitted that it was difficult to adjust to life as usual.

It's not surprising that her leg took some time to recover. In her final procedure, performed during her final days in the hospital, we had to seal the wound with a sixty-four-square-inch skin graft obtained from her thigh. "My little burn," she explained, rolling up the leg of her trousers to show me.

It wasn't attractive, but the wound looked really decent to me. It was around the size of my hand and extended from beneath her knee to her toes. Naturally, the skin colour was somewhat off, and the wound edges were piled up. The transplant also made her foot and ankle appear wider and bulkier. However, the wound did not have any exposed sections, as they sometimes do. And the grafted skin was soft and pliant, with no tightness, hardness, or contraction. Her grafted thigh was a vivid cherry red, but it was rapidly fading.

She had struggled to regain full use of her leg. When she initially arrived home, she was unable to stand since her muscles were weak and aching. Her leg would collapse right beneath her. When she regained her strength, she discovered she was still unable to walk. Nerve injury had caused a considerable foot drop. She saw Dr. Studdert, who warned her that this was something she might always have. After months of hard physical therapy, she was able to retrain herself to walk heel-toe. By the time I arrived, she was jogging. She'd also returned to work, this time as an assistant at the Hartford headquarters of a major insurance company.

A year later, Eleanor was still plagued by what had occurred to her. She still didn't know where the bacterium came from. Perhaps it was the foot bath and pedicure she received the day before the wedding at a modest hair and nail salon. Perhaps the grass outside the wedding reception hall, where she danced barefoot with a conga line. Perhaps someplace in her own home. She was terrified of cuts and fevers. She wouldn't go swimming. She refused to take a bath. She wouldn't even allow the water in the shower to reach her feet. Her family was planning a trip to Florida shortly, but the prospect of moving so far away from her doctors scared her.

The chances, the apparent unpredictability, were what bothered her the most. "First, they say the odds of you getting this are nothing—

one in two hundred fifty thousand," she told me. But then I understood it. Then they say the chances of me beating it are slim. And I defeated those odds." Now, when she asked our doctors if she could catch the flesh-eating bacteria again, we assured her that the odds are still improbably low, one in two hundred fifty thousand, the same as before.

That May, she did travel to Florida. It was windless and sweltering, and one day, off the eastern coast above Pompano, she dipped one bare foot into the ocean, then the other. Finally, despite her misgivings, Eleanor plunged in and went swimming in the ocean.

The contents of this book may not be copied, reproduced or transmitted without the express written permission of the author or publisher. Under no circumstances will the publisher or author be responsible or liable for any damages, compensation or monetary loss arising from the information contained in this book, whether directly or indirectly. .

Disclaimer Notice:

Although the author and publisher have made every effort to ensure the accuracy and completeness of the content, they do not, however, make any representations or warranties as to the accuracy, completeness, or reliability of the content. , suitability or availability of the information, products, services or related graphics contained in the book for any purpose. Readers are solely responsible for their use of the information contained in this book

Every effort has been made to make this book possible. If any omission or error has occurred unintentionally, the author and publisher will be happy to acknowledge it in upcoming versions.

Copyright © 2023

All rights reserved.

Printed in Great Britain
by Amazon